REFLEX EPILEPSY, BEHAVIORAL
THERAPY AND
CONDITIONAL REFLEXES

Publication Number 1006

AMERICAN LECTURE SERIES®

A Monograph in
The BANNERSTONE DIVISION *of*
AMERICAN LECTURES IN OBJECTIVE PSYCHIATRY

Edited by

WILLIAM HORSLEY GANTT, M.D.
Pavlovian Laboratory
Veterans Administration Hospital
Perry Point, Maryland

Reflex Epilepsy, Behavioral Therapy and Conditional Reflexes

By

FRANCIS M. FORSTER, M.D.

Detling Professor of Neurology and
Chairman of the Department
Center for Health Sciences
University of Wisconsin
Madison, Wisconsin

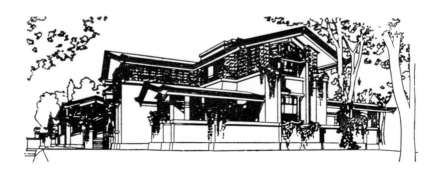

CHARLES C THOMAS · PUBLISHER
Springfield · Illinois · U.S.A.

Published and Distributed Throughout the World by
CHARLES C THOMAS • PUBLISHER

Bannerstone House
301-327 East Lawrence Avenue, Springfield, Illinois, U.S.A.

© 1977, by CHARLES C THOMAS • PUBLISHER
ISBN 0-398-03614-4
Library of Congress Catalog Card Number: 76-29659

Printed in the United States of America
W-2

Library of Congress Cataloging in Publication Data

Forster, Francis M.
    Reflex epilepsy, behavioral therapy, and conditional
reflexes.

    (American lecture series; publication No. 1006)
    Bibliography: p.
    Includes index.
    1. Epilepsy. 2. Behavior therapy. 3. Conditioned
response. I. Title. [DNLM: 1. Epilepsy—Therapy.
2. Behavior therapy. 3. Conditioning, Classical.
WL385 F733r]
RC372.F67   616.8'58   76-29659
ISBN 0-398-03614-4

THIS BOOK IS DEDICATED TO THE MEMORY OF

Doctor Hans H. Reese

1891-1973

Distinguished Neurologist,
Supportive Colleague,
and Devoted Friend

PREFACE

T HIS VOLUME IS the result of numerous influences by teachers, friends, and colleagues of many disciplines.

In my medical student and intern days in Cincinnati, Doctor A. R. Vonderahe encouraged me to seek a career in neurology. Through his auspices I came to the Neurological Unit at the Boston City Hospital. At that time, Doctor Tracy J. Putnam and Doctor H. Houston Merritt were in the process of discovering Dilantin®; Doctor and Mrs. Frederick Gibbs, working with Doctor William G. Lennox, were defining EEG correlates of seizure types; and Doctor Lennox was pursuing his historical and genetic studies in epilepsy. A Rockefeller Fellowship allowed me to spend a year in Doctor John F. Fulton's laboratory at Yale University. This was near the close of the era of the cortical ablation studies. Later, as a young faculty member at Jefferson Medical College, Doctor Bernard J. Alpers encouraged me to establish the EEG Laboratory and Epilepsy Clinic. Here it was that I saw my first cases of reflex epilepsy, and one of these cases (Case 1, Chapter 7) led to the exciting experience of collaborating with Doctor Wilder Penfield and Doctor Herbert H. Jasper.

In 1958, Doctor Pearce Bailey, Director of the National Institute of Neurological Diseases and Blindness, appointed me to chair the First Medical Exchange Mission to the USSR. The Pavlovian influence of Professor Simeon Sarkisov and Professor Vasili Zakusov, especially as interpreted and elaborated by my friend and colleague Doctor Paul Yakovlev, impressed me and led to the questions of possible etiologic association and therapeutic potentials between conditional reflexes and reflex epilepsy. This led inevitably to an association with Doctor W. Horsley Gantt and the late Professor Wulf Brogden. They reviewed my data, and Doctor Gantt especially has been encouraging and helpful in the area of interpretation throughout these years.

Many present and former members of the Department of Neurology at the University of Wisconsin are coauthors of the papers cited in this volume. Others who have advised and helped in the design and reporting of these studies are the late Doctor Hans H. Reese and Doctor Charles G. Matthews.

For these studies to come to a fruitful determination, much technical support was also necessary. The EEG technicians, Linda Meyer, Nancy Suchomel, Marjorie Bong, and Jeannette Patterson, throughout these years were especially helpful. Mr. Rolland Schultz, the electronic specialist, was helpful in so many ways, not the least being his expertise in cinematography. Ms. Mary Jeglum gave much needed help on the manuscript preparation.

The United States Public Health Service (USPHS) was generous in supporting this work under USPHS Grant NB-03360 awarded by the National Institute of Neurological Diseases and Blindness Council.

Help was also forthcoming from the private sector of the economy. For example, Otarion Hearing Aid Company made available the special eyeglasses for maintenance of conditioning. The computer automation described in Chapter 13 was acquired through the generous and anonymous contributions of industrialists in Madison, Wisconsin. Various radio stations and their announcers were of inestimable help in studying the patient with voice-induced epilepsy. Not only local stations, but also the networks, were of assistance in tracing musical programs which evoked seizures in our musicogenic patients.

In retrospect then, this work is the result of teachers and mentors, supporting personnel, public funding, and the help of the free enterprise system of our great country.

F.M.F.

CONTENTS

REFLEX EPILEPSY, BEHAVIORAL THERAPY AND CONDITIONAL REFLEXES

CHAPTER 1

EPILEPSY AND REFLEX EPILEPSY

E PILEPSY, ONE OF the oldest known diseases of mankind, was mentioned in the ancient writings of Hippocrates and others. For millenia there was confusion as to the nature of epilepsy. Various cultures attributed the condition to different etiologic factors, usually based upon superstitions. Temkin[1] reviewed these older concepts in his history of epilepsy, and set the milestone or landmark for modern scientific understanding of epilepsy in 1857, when Hughlings Jackson[2] defined epilepsy as the sudden excessive disorderly discharge of the grey matter of the brain. Concurrently the anatomists and physiologists of the late nineteenth and early twentieth centuries demonstrated the presence of electrical activity of the nervous system and the electrical excitability of the brain of animals. These latter observations led to the concept of cortical localization. These basic science contributions have recently been reviewed by Brazier.[3]

In the mid 1930s Hans Berger[4] demonstrated the presence of electrical activity of the brain of man and also showed that abnormalities occurred in this activity during seizures. This therefore substantiated Jackson's hypothesis of disorderly discharge, and extended it still further by demonstrating that the abnormal discharge is electrical in nature.

It is now known that these abnormal discharges may (a) arise from and be restricted to a particular area of the cerebral cortex, (b) spread from a particular area by cortical networks or transcortical pathways including the commisures, (c) spread from one area of cortex to the subcortical synchronizing networks and return as a generalized cortical discharge, as demonstrated by the atypical bilateral wave and spike dysrhythmias, or (d) originate in the subcortical synchronizing networks—the so-called centrencephalic seizures of Penfield and Jasper.[5]

3

Therapeutic processes may be aimed at removing or inhibiting the focal discharging cortex, or at inhibiting the spread of the abnormal discharge along the various pathways noted above. As shown in Chapter 15, the conditioning process results in alterations of these factors.

An intriguing and perplexing problem in epilepsy is the mechanism of triggering seizures. Why do some patients have multiple seizures in a day, others one in a day, a month, a year, or even less frequently? Given a discharging lesion, a brain with dysrhythmia, what precipitates the seizures at a particular time in the individual patient? Lennox[6] demonstrated some mechanisms in his Reservoir Theory, with the input of various metabolic, emotional, and other factors filling the reservoir until the dam (seizure threshold) overflows and a seizure results. A fundamental question in the given patient is, what precipitates his seizures?

The study of patients with sensory-evoked or reflex epilepsy is ideal in this regard. These patients, when presented with a stimulus, specific for the given patient, respond with a seizure. Marshall Hall[7] first described these cases as "reflex epilepsy." However, his description was not clear and involved also the spinal reflexes later to be well clarified by Sir Charles Sherrington.

Daube[8] concluded from his extensive review of the literature on sensory-precipitated seizures that the stimuli may be due to certain changes of sensory input, such as a sudden change of light; they may be rhythmical, such as repeated photic stimulation; and finally, they may be complex mental stimuli, such as in musicogenic epilepsy.

Certain well-documented instances of reflex epilepsy were reported in the older literature, such as the description by Hughlings Jackson[9] of a boy who had seizures when he was briskly tapped on the head. But the term "reflex epilepsy" fell into disuse as the literature became cluttered with confusing reports. Such reports attributed reflex epilepsy to eating habits, masturbation, intestinal parasites, and similar nondescript factors. Because of this confusion, the term "reflex epilepsy" has not been used as extensively during the past few decades as the more precise physiological term "sensory-evoked epilepsy." However, some forms of reflex epilepsy are not, in the usual sense, induced by sensory stimuli.

The studies related in this book demonstrate that higher cognitive functions play a role in some of the evoked epilepsies. The dissemination and acquisition of knowledge, memory patterns, anticipation of stimulus, the concept of stimulus, even decision making are cognitive functions which in this volume are found to play a role in reflex epilepsy. Since in a significant number of patients with reflex epilepsy, the seizures can be evoked by such higher cognitive functions rather than by simple sensory stimulation, the author has chosen to return to the term "reflex epilepsy."

At this point, the question might be asked: How important is reflex epilepsy? This question can be approached from several viewpoints; the incidence, the importance to the involved patients, and the possibilty of the study of reflex epilepsy serving as a tool or guide for further observations in epilepsy.

In regard to the incidence of reflex epilepsy, Symonds[10] found sensory evocation played a part in 6.5 percent of 1000 cases of epilepsy. Servit[11] reported an evoking factor in 5 percent of 895 epileptic patients. Thus, roughly 5 to 6 percent of epileptic patients could have an evoking factor. The incidence of epilepsy according to the older studies of Lennox was 0.5 percent of the general population. This figure was based on World Wars I and II draft figures. However, more recent epidemiologic studies would suggest that the incidence is closer to 1 percent. This would result in a figure of two million epileptics in the United States. If 5 percent have some evoking factor, this would indicate a potential population of 100,000 patients in this country with reflex epilepsy.

The importance of reflex epilepsy to the individual patient is quite obvious. The evoking stimuli are present in everyday life and, for the most part, are beyond the control of the patient. Moreover, the reflex epilepsies, as noted by many authors, are very frequently refractory to drug therapy, and many of them are not appropriate for surgical therapy. Other modes of treatment, including behavioral, are indicated.

The importance of observations on reflex epilepsy for the

further understanding of epilepsy in general is quite clear. The predictable evocation of seizures creates a situation conducive to controlled studies. These studies, as developed in later chapters, show that the evoked dysrhythmias can be altered or abolished by means of behavioral techniques. The clinical and neurophysiological changes are indeed significant and may lead to broader application in the total field of epilepsy.

GENERAL ASPECTS OF CASE FINDING

The presence of reflex epilepsy may be ascertained either through a case history or by laboratory examination. In case finding, the history is most important and has the highest yield. It is important to listen carefully as the patient and the family describe the situations in which seizures occur. All too frequently the physician brushes over the casual observation by the family that the patient has seizures almost every morning upon walking out the front door of the house on the way to school; or the comment that the patient has all or almost all of the seizures on certain days of the week, and especially at certain hours. These questions should lead one to further interrogations. Do those early morning seizures occur on bright sunny days? Does the house face east? What is the patient doing during the certain hours on weekdays—listening to a particular radio program or watching a particular TV program? Does the patient experiencing seizures while watching TV have them with "flop-over" (photic) or while looking at the focusing panel (pattern) prior to the onset of the program? The mother who noted that her child had a seizure every time she dropped a dish on the floor or someone rapped on the kitchen door unexpectedly had long ago made the diagnosis of startle epilepsy.

Musicogenic epilepsy in a given patient is not usually diagnosed as being attributed to music for a considerable period of time, and then it is usually a member of the family who makes the deduction of the relationship of music to the occurrence of seizures.

Many of the somatosensory-evoked seizures are so obviously related to discrete and readily observable stimuli that the diagnosis is made early. The obvious stimulus may take the form of a sudden blow to a part of the body, and the seizure which follows usually results in falling. These two events are sufficiently dramatic to provide sufficient basis for an early diagnosis.

It is important to obtain relevant information from the family and the patient. If they do not volunteer, one must ask specifically, in all cases of epilepsy, if the patient or family are aware of any precipitating factors which might cause the seizure. No possibility, however remote, of a reflex cause should be overlooked. If at all possible, the precise sequence of events should be reconstructed in the EEG laboratory.

Patients suspected of having reflex epilepsy are best studied under constant audiovisual monitoring with split-screen technique. This makes possible the recording of the image of the patient on one half of the screen and of the EEG tracings on the other half, while the audio channel carries a continuous record of the auditory stimuli and events in the environment. Replaying in slow motion or regular timing allows for the study of the entire sequence and for correlations of audiovisual environmental changes with the clinical changes in the patient and any electroencephalographic concomitants.

In the Epilepsy Center at the University of Wisconsin Health Sciences Center, laboratory personnel have striven to reconstruct the situation in which seizures occurred. No suggestion on the part of the patient was too ridiculous to cast in a scene. By following this principle, the usual and the unusual forms of reflex epilepsy reported in this volume were determined and studied.

Not all patients referred for reflex epilepsy were found to have this entity. The occurrence of a clinical event in response to a sensory stimulus does not in itself establish the diagnosis of reflex epilepsy. The event must be a truly epileptic one. Pseudoseizures, hyperventilation syndrome, and neurologic entities other than epileptic occurred in patients suspected of known kinds of reflex epilepsy. In Chapter 11, the differential diagnosis of various forms of reflex epilepsy is discussed in detail.

It is also necessary to determine whether or not spontaneous dysrhythmias and/or seizures occur. That is, do seizures or dysrhythmias occur without the presence of evoking stimuli? It is therefore necessary to have a recording of sufficient duration in the resting state to ascertain if this phenomenon is present. EEG recording in the awake state and during sensory restriction is also useful for this purpose. To achieve sensory restriction, the patients are either placed in a darkened soundproof chamber or in the research laboratory and wear black goggles and earphones which deliver a white noise. This state is maintained for twenty to thirty minutes, and the patient is kept awake by touch when necessary. Many patients with sensory-evoked epilepsy have some spontaneous dysrhythmia. It is necessary to document that the reflex dysrhythmia is invariably evoked by the stimulus and is not merely a fortuitous concurrence of spontaneous dysrhythmia and stimulation.

The diagnosis of reflex epilepsy depends upon the demonstration of the repeated and predictable occurrence of dysrhythmia or dysrhythmia and seizures in response to a particular stimulus. It should be noted that in some of the more complex types, especially in the auditory-evoked seizures, definite EEG responses could not be evoked in the laboratory. However, most if not all of the patients' multiple seizures related only to the precipitating stimulus, thus eliminating the possibility of chance. The single occurrence of discharge or seizure with the presentation of the stimulus is certainly not sufficient to warrant the diagnosis of reflex epilepsy. A spontaneous dysrhythmia or seizure could easily have occurred at that time.

The author and his colleagues have not had the opportunity to study all existing forms of reflex epilepsy. Some of the forms not yet seen are considered in the chapters relevant to them. For example, in the chapter on somatosensory-evoked epilepsy, reported instances of seizures due to immersion and to coitus are discussed.

There are other reported instances of reflex epilepsy which cannot readily be placed in the categories herein described. Seizures have been induced by vestibular stimulation, using the caloric method. This was first reported by Marie and Pierre[12] and later by Jones.[13] Studies, after the advent of EEG, by Behrman and Wyke[14] and Orban and Lang[15] confirmed that caloric stimulation may activate temporal lobe EEG foci. Doudomopoulis,[16] working in the author's laboratory at Georgetown, was unable to confirm the findings of EEG activation of temporal lobe foci by caloric stimulation, and such cases have not been seen at the University of Wisconsin.

Evocation of seizures by olfactory stimuli is exceedingly rare. This was described by Gowers,[17] and Stevens[18] reported an increase in EEG spiking in patients with temporal lobe foci when they were administered olfactory stimuli. No such case has been studied at the University of Wisconsin.

The role of emotional or mental stimuli requires careful study. It is hoped that with the background of these detailed studies on the effect of readily measurable stimuli and of definite but elusive stimuli, especially in the higher cognitive functions, as recounted in this volume, it will be possible to proceed methodically to the study of the role of emotional and mental stimuli in evoking seizures.

Since 1961, seventy-three cases of reflex epilepsy have been studied in detail at the University of Wisconsin. In addition, a large number of patients thought possibly to have reflex epilepsy have been studied but were diagnosed as having other conditions. Therefore, in Chapter 11 which deals with the differential diagnosis of epilepsy, some of the more illustrative cases representing conditions other than, but easily confused with, reflex epilepsy are examined.

TABLE 1

CASES OF REFLEX EPILEPSY STUDIED

Kinds of Reflex Epilepsy	*Number of Cases*
Visually induced	39
Auditory-evoked	10
Musicogenic	5
Language/reading	11*
Decision-making	2*
Movement-induced	1
Somatosensory	4
Associated with eating	2
	73

* One patient appears in both series.

Table I presents the number of cases of reflex epilepsy in each major group. The observations made on these patients, the conclusions drawn from the observations, and the innovative mode of therapy introduced are the basis for this book.

REFERENCES

1. Temkin, Owsei: *The Falling Sickness. A History of Epilepsy from the Greeks to the Beginnings of Modern Neurology.* Baltimore, Johns Hopkins, 1945, pp. xv; 380.
2. Jackson, J. Hughlings: A study of convulsions. *Trans St. Andrews Med Grad Assn, 3:*1-45, 1870. Reprinted in Taylor, J. (Ed.): *Selected Writings of John Hughlings Jackson.* London, Houghton and Stoughton, 1931.
3. Brazier, M. B., M.A.B.: The search for the neuronal mechanisms in epilepsy: An overview. *Neurology, 24:*903, 1974.
4. Berger, Hans: Uber die Entstehung der Erscheinungen des grossen epileptischen, Anfalls. *Klin Wochenschr, 14:*217, 1935.
5. Penfield, Wilder and Jasper, Herbert H.: *Epilepsy and the Functional Anatomy of the Brain.* Boston, Little, Brown, 1954, pp. xv, 896.
6. Lennox, W. G.: *Science and Seizures.* 2nd ed. New York and London, Harper, 1946, pp. xi, 258.
7. Hall, Marshall: *Synopsis of the Spinal System.* London, J. Mallett, 1850, p. 100.
8. Daube, J.: Precipitated seizures. A review. *J Nerv Ment Dis, 141:*524, 1965.
9. Jackson, J. Hughlings: Fits following touching the head. *Lancet, 1:*274, 1895.
10. Symonds, C.: Excitation and inhibitition in epilepsy. *Brain, 82:*133, 1959.
11. Servit, Z., Machek, J., and Stercova, A.: Reflex influences in pathogenesis of epilepsy. In: *Reflex Mechanisms in the Genesis of Epilepsy.* Amsterdam, Elsevier, 1963, p. 107.
12. Marie, P. and Pierre, J.: Etude sur la variabilite des reactions vestibulaired des epileptiques etudes par la methode de barany. *Rev Neurol, 29:*86, 1922.
13. Jones, I.: Neuro-otologic studies in epilepsy. *JAMA, 81:*2083, 1923.
14. Behrman, S. and Wyke, B.: Vestibulogenic seizures. *Brain, 84:*529, 1958.
15. Orban, L. and Lang, J.: Zur Pathogenese der vestibulogenen Epilepsie, *Psychiat Neurol, 146:*193, 1963.

16. Doudoumopoulis, A. N.: The electroencephalogram in stimulation of the labyrinth. *Bulletin Georgetown University Medical Center,* 9:173, 1955.
17. Gowers, W.: *Epilepsy and Other Chronic Convulsive Diseases.* New York, W. Wood, 1885.
18. Stevens, J.: Central and peripheral factors in epileptic discharge. *Arch Neurol,* 7:330, 1962.

CHAPTER 2

EPILEPSY EVOKED BY VISUAL STIMULI

T HE CATEGORY OF visually induced seizures includes the oldest known and the most frequently occurring form of reflex epilepsy, namely seizures induced by intermittent light. This form is usually referred to as photoconvulsive or photosensitive epilepsy, and is sometimes called photogenic epilepsy. However, presentations of other visual stimuli may evoke seizures. The various kinds of visually induced reflex epilepsy known at the present time consist of seizures evoked by:

—Intermittent light (stroboscopic stimulation)
—Viewing patterns
—Eye closure
—Viewing certain objects
—Viewing certain colors

The vast majority of patients with visually induced seizures are in the first group; that is, their seizures are induced by flashing lights. Celesia[1] found that 4.3 percent of 1,835 epileptic patients were photoconvulsive. The listing above is in the order of frequency of occurrence. The last two forms, object- and color-induced are indeed rare. The various kinds of visually induced epilepsy also occur in combinations as are noted below.

Visually induced seizures were known in ancient Greece. According to Lennox,[2] potential slaves about to be purchased, in order to determine if they were epileptic, were exposed to the rotations of a potter's wheel in a bright light.

In ancient times, seizures were also described as occurring upon viewing a horrible sight, but it is possible that these were syncopal attacks, with some twitching as occurs in the various vasovagal syncopies. (cf. Case 4, Chapter 11) In 1881, Gowers[3] commented that bright light could precipitate myoclonic or petit mal seizures, and in 1882, Ranney[4] noted seizures precipitated by changes in light intensity and by reflection of light from rough water. In 1927, Holmes[5] stated that the viewing of a movie could induce seizures. Flickering was a prominent feature of early movies. Cobb,[6] in 1947, described flicker as a significant factor in visual precipitation of seizures. Gastaut,[7, 8] Bickford and his colleagues,[9] and others[10, 11, 12] have written extensively on photosensitivity.

The seizures induced by flicker stimulation are usually minor seizures of the petit mal type, although major motor seizures may occur. In the University of Wisconsin study series, only three patients each had a single major motor seizure induced in the laboratory. This was accidental, as there was no attempt made at any time to induce a major motor seizure. On several occasions, prolonged petit mal seizures (which the family called convulsions) were witnessed. The seizures were, however, characterized by generalized clonic movements occurring in synchrony with an atypical three per second wave and spike bisynchrony. Some automatisms may also occur during the course of the minor motor seizures.

Alterations of the EEG induced by intermittent light stimulation are of two types: (a) photo myoclonus and (b) photoconvulsive. Photo myoclonus (Fig. 1) is not considered an epileptic phenomenon but rather muscle artifact recorded from the scalp muscles. It begins with the onset of stimulation and ceases when the stroboscopic stimulation ends. Since this is not considered to be truly epileptic, no cases of photo myoclonus were included in the series.

The photoconvulsive response (Fig. 2) is quite characteristic and definitely epileptic. The cerebral dysrhythmia is usually of the atypical spike and wave type. The slow wave may be somewhat faster or slower than three per second, and there are usually multiple polyphasic spikes. Frequently there is a cortical area from which the dysrhythmia first seems to arise. This may be frontal or, more frequently, occipital. Dysrhythmia, when well developed, persists after cessation of the stroboscopic stimulation. Presumbaly this dysrhythmia is either a primary or, more frequently, a secondary bisynchrony. It is either a

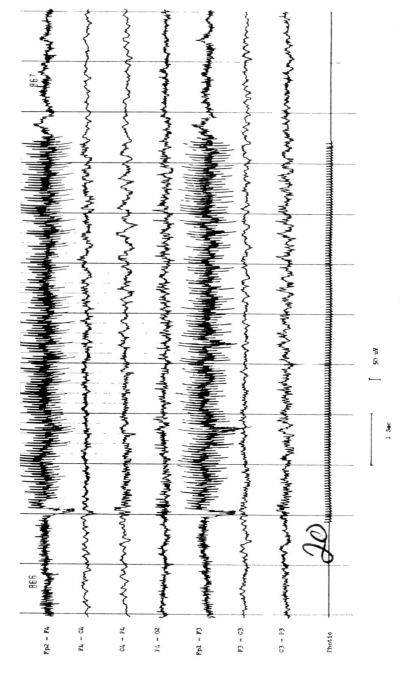

Figure 1. EEG during photomyoclonus. No specific EEG changes. Note EMG predominately frontal, coinciding in onset and cessation with photic stimulation.

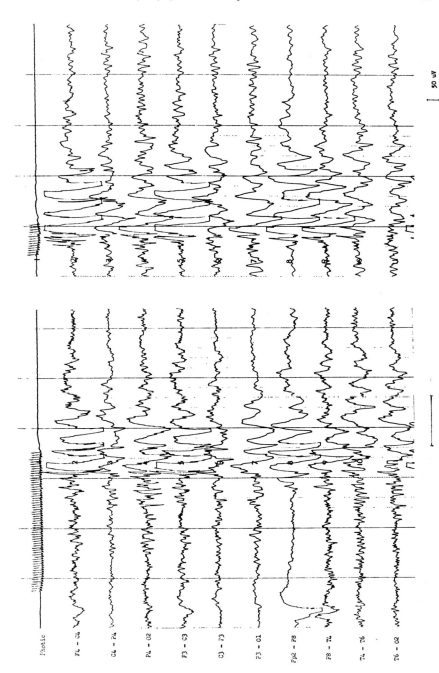

Figure 2.   Photosensitivity.   Atypical spike-wave dysrhythmia evoked by photic stimulation.

primary firing from the reticular formation or a primary firing from a focal cortical area into the reticular formation and a return firing of the entire hemispheres (secondary bisynchrony).

Photic-induced seizures occur at a particular frequency range for a given patient. These frequencies may vary from single individual flashes to flicker fusion point, but they are usually between ten to thirty-five per second and more usually between fifteen to twenty-five cycles per second. The range of stroboscopic frequency which evokes the photoconvulsive responses is quite constant for a given patient, although he may show some slight variations from day to day.

In the laboratory, a series of thirty-nine cases of visually induced epilepsy have been studied. Patients were referred or selected because visual stimuli evoked major motor seizures or frequent minor (petit mal) seizures. All patients in this series were studied in the standardized fashion as described below.

STANDARDIZED TESTING FOR VISUALLY INDUCED EPILEPSY

In all patients suspected of visually induced epilepsy, certain baseline studies were obtained to determine the presence or absence of spontaneously occurring dysrhythmias. The baseline studies consisted of EEGs in the resting state, during hyperventilation, whenever possible in the sleep state, and in the sensory-deprived state.

The results of photic stimulation (Fig. 3) were studied systematically, and the entire procedure was AV taped for replay study. The patient was placed at a standard distance from an opaque screen (36 inches) behind which was the (Grass) stroboscope flanked by two photoflood bulbs. These photoflood bulbs were the only sources of ambient light in the laboratory while the patient was being studied. The current for these photofloods passed through a rheostat so that the ambient light levels could be varied from 0 to 600 footcandles at the bridge of the patient's nose. However, during the studies, the ambient light was decreased to the point where a reasonable image of the patient appeared on the AV monitor screen during stimulation.

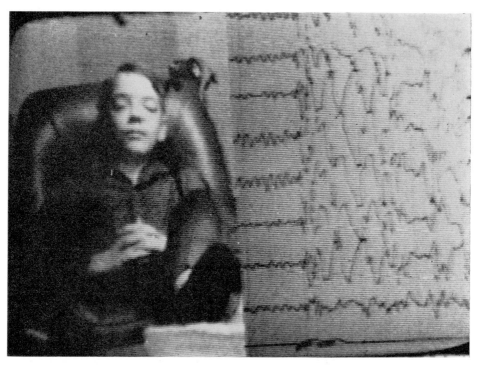

Figure 3. From AV tape recording. Patient's eyes closed in myoclonic jerk. Stroboscopic stimulation indicated on bottom channel of EEG. Atypical spike-wave dysrhythmia evoked by stimulation. Case 35.

The specific flicker frequency which induced seizure discharges was carefully ascertained for each patient. The flash rate was started with single flashes, then with bursts of one per second flashes lasting three to ten seconds. The frequency was gradually increased and administered in bursts until the lower limit of the dysrhythmia-producing flicker was ascertained. Stimulations were then begun at flicker fusion, and gradually decreased in frequency until the upper level of the range was determined. Sampling was then made at three to five cycles per second variations between the lower and upper limits. If for example, the lowest frequency that evoked dysrhythmia was fifteen per second and the highest thirty-five per second, samples were made at 19, 23, 28, and 32 per second frequencies.

It is important to begin the search for the evoking stimulus range beyond the sensitive range and gradually approach it. If one begins in the center, for example, at twenty per second, and proceeds in both directions in a patient who is sensitive between twelve and twenty-five per second, the boundaries can be falsely extended, by the conditioning factor at work in the testing, to eight or nine per second at the lower end of the range and to twenty-eight to thirty-two per second at the upper end. These false boundaries are dependent upon the conditioning factor.

The critical flicker frequency was studied with eyes opened and eyes closed. There does not appear to be any significant difference in the flicker rate that evoked seizures in the same patient between eyes opened and eyes closed conditions, but some patients are not sensitive at all with eyes opened (Fig. 4); others are insensitive with eyes closed. The degree of sensitivity may also be greater in either of these conditions.

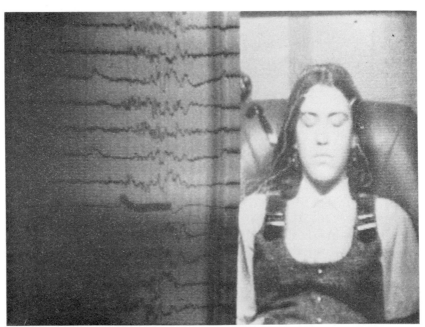

Figure 4. From AV tape recording. Shows photosensitivity with eyes closed. This patient had no dysrhythmia evoked when her eyes were open. Case 18.

The minimum strobe intensity necessary to evoke a dysrhythmia was determined in the course of the scanning for frequencies. The testing began with the lowest intensity and if, in the first scanning for frequencies, no dysrhythmia occurred, the intensity was increased by one step and the process repeated. Thus the minimum strobe intensity was determined. The ambient light, of course, plays a role, for there is a reciprocal relationship between the intensity of the stroboscope and of the room light. However, some ambient light was necessary for AV recording.

Many photosensitive patients are monocularly insensitive[13, 14] (Figs. 5A and 5B). This is determined by patching one eye. The usual ophthalmologist's eye shade is insufficient for this purpose. Most satisfactory is a patch of soft black velvet, molded across the eye from forehead to cheek and held in place by the patient's hand. Special care is necessary to have the bridge of the nose covered by the middle or index and middle fingers over the velvet. A slight light leak during stimulations can change monocular insensitivity to monocular sensitivity, at least for a time. This again is a conditioning process. When one eye was satisfactorily patched, several series of stimulations within the noxious range were administered. The process was then repeated after the patch had been changed to the other eye.

The effect of strobe-to-patient distance was not uniformly studied, for this equation is but another expression of intensity. The farther the distance, the less the intensity. The distance was kept constant for these studies.

Colored filters have not been used extensively in this study. While it has been reported that certain colors, especially red, may decrease sensitivity, this has not been uniform and in fact, in some patients, it has been reported that red flashes are more noxious to the patient.[15] However, in the few instances wherein filters were used, and it seemed that a red filter appeared to decrease the patient's sensitivity to the flickering light, a check for intensity showed that the filter had decreased the intensity. When the intensity of the red flickering was brought up to the minimum evoking intensity of the unfiltered stroboscopic stimulations, the dysrhythmia reappeared. For these determinations, an accurate footcandle light meter was employed.

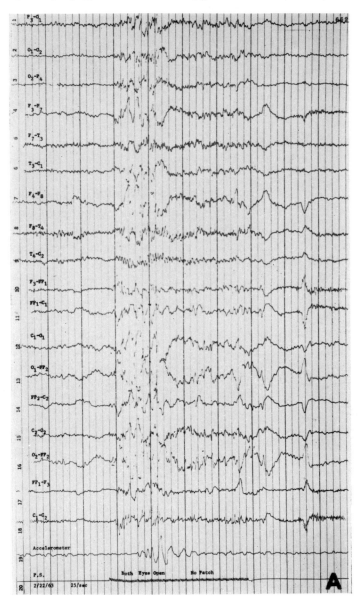

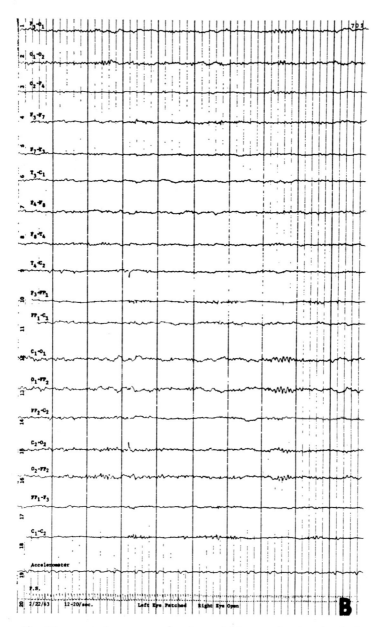

Figure 5. Demonstrates monocular insensitivity to photic stimulation. In 5A stimulus administered with both eyes open. Photic stimulations between 15 and 35 cycles per second evoked dysrhythmia. In 5B photic stimulation with vision of one eye occluded by velvet patch failed to evoke dysrhythmia. Case 1. Reprinted from *Epilepsia*, 5:156, 1964.

Patients who were self-stimulators were asked to induce attacks in the laboratory. The ambient light was increased to 600 footcandles and the patients were asked to wave their fingers before their eyes. A photoelectric cell was placed on the forehead, and it recorded the self-induced flashes along with the EEG. When the patients succeeded in self-stimulation, they usually achieved at least ten per second stimulations (Fig. 6).

To determine the presence or absence of pattern sensitivity, various patterns were presented. The patterns described by Bickford[16, 17] were employed. These consist of vertical lines sharply drawn in black and white, similar horizontal lines, and screen grids. To these patterns a checkered table cloth pattern, a series of curving lines, and radiating "sunburst" were added. Also, specific objects which had evoked seizures in the particular patient at home were brought to the laboratory and incorporated into the array of stimulus material.

In the direct method of pattern presentation, these patterns were held momentarily over the EEG to document them on AV tape and then presented in a bright light to the patient with eyes closed. Upon command the patient opened his/her eyes, stared at the pattern for 10 seconds, then closed the eyes, whereupon the pattern was removed and the next pattern presented.

The patterns were also presented indirectly by projection on a screen before the patient. A Super 8® cassette movie projector was used, and the patterns were seen on the screen projected in front of the patient. This allowed a more standardized method of the presentation of the pattern.

Even when the presentation of a pattern appeared to evoke a dysrhythmia, this was not sufficient evidence to determine pattern sensitivity. That particular pattern was then presented repeatedly, but with the interjection of other patterns and pictures. The evocation had to be invariably associated with the particular pattern or patterns.

Once pattern sensitivity was definitely established, the effect of monocular presentations was studied. Here it was not necessary to be so exact in blocking out light; the use of an ophthalmologist's patch sufficed. However, it was simpler for the patient to continue in the same manner with the velvet patch.

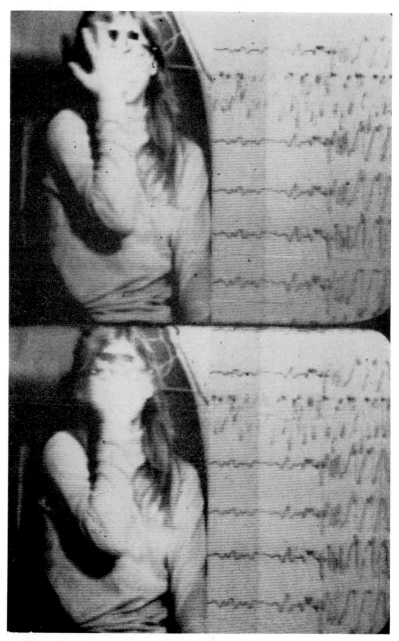

Figure 6. Patient, self-stimulating by finger-waving in laboratory and evoking seizure. Patch on forehead contains photoelectric cell. Second channel of EEG records from the photoelectric cell and shows the rate of stimulation. Atypical spike-wave dysrhythmia seen in other channels.

Eye closure as a source of dysrhythmia or seizures is not common but should be tested routinely in the patient with visually induced epilepsy. This is simple to do. In the study, the ambient light was increased to the maximum available in the laboratory (600 footcandles) and the patient instructed to open and to close his/her eyes, not in a rhythmic fashion but on command. If dysrhythmia occurred on eye closure in the bright light, the commands were repeated with the patient in virtual darkness. This was to determine whether the evoking sensory stimulus was visual or proprioceptive. The effect of monocular patching upon eye closure evocation was also observed.

Since the description in Case 39 of epilepsy evoked by viewing a certain color,[18] the introduction of colors was added to the testing procedure. This was accomplished by showing the patients, in serial fashion, a number of color swatches such as are used to select paints. Their EEGs were observed while they identified each color as correctly as possible and noted whether or not they liked it. In no other patient was color-evoked dysrhthymia found.

CLINICAL AND LABORATORY OBSERVATIONS

A total of thirty-nine patients were studied in this series of visually-evoked epileptics. The overall data on thirty-eight patients is presented in Table II. Case 39 is presented later and in detail because of the rarity of color/object-induced epilepsy. The various kinds of visually induced epilepsy and the combinations of the types studied are presented in Table III. The various clinical and laboratory features of these different kinds of visually induced epilepsy are now reviewed.

Photic-induced Epilepsy

Thirty-four cases of photic-induced epilepsy were studied. Twenty-one of these patients had only photic-induced seizures. Ten patients had, in addition, seizures evoked by patterns. Two patients had seizures evoked by photic and eye closure stimuli. Only one patient had dysrhythmias evoked by photic, pattern, and eye closure stimuli.

In the laboratory series of thirty-four patients with photosensitivity, the preponderance of females over males is significant

TABLE II

Case #	Sex	Age	Age of Onset	Seizure Type	Family History	Intelligence	Other Diseases	Freq. Range	Photic Sensitivity				Eye Closure	Spon. Dys.	Self-Induction
									Mon-ocular	E.O.	E.C.	Pattern Sensitivity			
1	F	21	18	PM & MM	Brother with syncope	College Graduate	0	15 - 35	0	+	+	0	0	0	0
2	F	12	9	PM & MM	Brother with seizures - ? photic	IQ 86	0	15 - 45	0	+	+	0	0	+	+
3	F	5	Infancy	Myoclonic	0	Severe M.R.	Trisomy-D Anomaly	1 - 50	+	+	+	0	0	+	+
4	M	13	7	PM & MM	Post-traumatic seizures in 1 aunt	7th grade		10 - 16	0	+	+	0	0	+	0
5	M	22	6	PM	Sister with seizures	IQ 101	0	10 - 30	0	+	+	0	0	0	0
6	F	13	5	PM & MM	0	IQ 97	0	10 - 20	+	+	+	0	0	0	0
7	M	10	8 mo.	PM & MM	Adopted ?	IQ 80	0	12 - 16	0	+	+	0	0	+	0
8	F	6	4	PM	0	MA 3½	Behavior disorder	6 - 35	0	+	+	0	0	0	0
9	M	18	6	PM & MM	Brothers	IQ 97	0	15 - 30	0	+	+	0	0	+	0
10	M	18	6	PM & MM	Brothers	IQ 95	0	15 - 30	0	+	+	0	0	+	0
11	M	16	12	PM	0	IQ 99	0	15 - 20	0	+	+	0	0	+	0
12	F	12	3	PM & MM	Sibling with febrile seizures	IQ 74	0	10 - 25	0	+	+	0	0	+	+
13	F	13	12	PM	Negative	11 H.S.	0	12.5 - 30	0	+	0	0	0	0	0
14	F	19	10	PM & MM	Maternal cousin with seizures	IQ 113	0	13 - 30	0	+	+	0	0	0	-

TABLE II (cont.)

Case No.	Sex	Age	Age of Onset	Seizure Type	Family History	Intelli-gence	Other Diseases	Photic Sensitivity				Pattern Sensitivity	Eye Closure	Spon. Dys.	Self-Induction
								Freq. Range	Mon-ocular	E.O.	E.C.				
15	F	12	9	PM & MM	Father has MM seizures	Normal	0	10 - 13 20 - 22	0	+	+	0	0	+	+
16	F	17	13	PM & MM	0	IQ 99	0	19 - 20	R. eye only	+	+	0	0	0	+
17	F	21	14	MM & PM	Brother with seizures	IQ 118	0	17 - 19	0	+	0	0	0	0	0
18	F	16	12	PM & MM	0	11 H.S.	0	11 - 12	0	0	+	0	0	+	0
19	F	10	3	PM	Paternal uncle with childhood seizures	MA 4	Equino varus	8 - 35	0	+	+	0	0	+	+
20	M	6	5	MM & PM	0	IQ 91	Cerebral palsy	20 - 25	0	+	+	0	0	+	0
21	M	23	17	MM & myoclonic	Mother also had cerebellar degeneration	IQ 85	Cerebellar degeneration	6 - 30	+	+	+	0	0	+	0
22	M	18	13	Myoclonic	0	College Grad.	0	17 - 20	0	+	+	+	0	0	0
23	M	17						17 - 55	0	+	+	+	0	0	0
24	F	24	12	MM & PM	0	College Grad.	0	20 - 35	+	+	+	+	0	+	0
25	F	11	6	PM & MM	Paternal uncle with seizures	Dull-N	Head injury age 2	14 - 16	0	+	0	+	0		
26	F	16	2	PM & MM		IQ 52	Cerebellar degeneration	10 - 35	0	+		+	0	+	+
27	F	13	3	PM & MM	Paternal cousin with seizures	IQ 63	0	15 - 20	0	+	+	+	0	+	+

TABLE II (cont.)

Case No.	Sex	Age	Age of Onset	Seizure Type	Family History	Intelligence	Other Diseases	Photic Sensitivity				Pattern Sensitivity	Eye Closure	Spon. Dys.	Self-Induction
								Freq. Range	Mon-ocular	E.O.	E.C.				
28	F	39	14	MM & PM	Paternal uncle and 1 sibling	H.S. ed	0	15 - 40	0	+	0	+	0	0	0
29	F	19	8	PM & MM	0	11 Coll student	0	13 - 45	0	+	+	+	0	0	0
30	F	12	8	PM & MM	Mother had seizures	7th grade	0	8 - 24	0	+	+	+	0	0	+
31	F	13	1	PM & MM	0	IQ 109	0	16 - 18	0	+	+	+	0	+	+
32	F	9	½	PM & MM	Paternal cousin with febrile seizures	IQ 39	0	0	0	+	0	+	0	+	?
33	F	7	1	PM & MM	0	IQ 55	0	0	0	+	0	+	0	+	+
34	F	2	4 mo.	PM & MM	0	Retarded	Otitis	0	0	+	0	+	0		+
35	M	12		PM & MM	0	N	0	13 - 30	0	+	+	0	+	+	0
36	F	14	10	PM & MM	Uncle with seizures	Dull N	0	15 - 20	0	+	+	0	+	+	0
37	F	19	18	MM & PM	Paternal and maternal cousins with seizures	IQ 88	Schizophrenic	0				0	+	0	0
38	F	23	0	0	0	IQ 93	M.S.	12.5 - 15	0	+	+	+	+	0	0

TABLE III

NUMBER OF CASES AND KINDS OF VISUALLY INDUCED
EPILEPSY STUDIED

Photic	Pattern	Eye Closure	Color/Object
21	—	—	—
10	10	—	—
—	3	—	—
2	—	2	—
1	1	1	—
—	—	1	—
—	—	—	1
34	14	4	1

(23:11). The higher prevalence among females has been noted before; the process was considered to be "more malignant"[19] in the female. This latter observation has not been the experience in this study as no significant difference in severity was noted between males and females.

The ages noted are the age at which the patient was studied in the laboratory. The age of onset was, of course, much earlier in most of them. The rarity of the condition in older patients is noticeable, for there were only four patients past the age of twenty years. Most remarkable was the woman aged thirty-nine years who was still photosensitive. Ehret and Schneider[20] observed an older patient who for thirty-two years had self-induced seizures.

The rate of flicker fusion that evoked the seizures varied considerably, but the fifteen to twenty per second flashes evoked seizures in almost all of the patients. The range extended from a very narrow range in two patients of 12.5 to 15 per second to an extensive range of 6 to 35 per second. Case 3, with a range of less than one per second to fifty per second was a markedly retarded, malformed, five-year-old, one-eyed, trisomy-D- anomaly patient. The patient's only voluntary activity was covering her one eye with her fist and uncovering it in order to evoke myoclonic jerks.

In describing the technique of studying the patients, it was noted that samplings were made in the frequency band between the lowest and highest flicker frequencies which evoked seizures.

In all patients but one (Case 15), the stimulations throughout the entire band of sensitivity evoked seizures. This individual patient had two separate narrow bands, one between ten and thirteen, and the other between twenty and twenty-two. Stimulations at these frequencies evoked seizures, but stimulations in the intervening band (fourteen to nineteen per second) did not.

When the same frequencies which had evoked seizures and dysrhythmia upon binocular presentation were presented monocularly, seizures and dysrhythmia seldom appeared (in only four of thirty-four photosensitive cases). In only one patient, Case 16, was there monocular sensitivity with only one eye. She had dysrhythmia evoked when the appropriate flicker frequency was presented to the right eye only, but not when presented to the left eye only.

One patient when stimulated had dysrhythmia only when her eyes were closed and had normal responses when her eyes were open (Case 18). Four patients had dysrhythmia only when stimulated with their eyes open but not when closed.

In this series of thirty-four cases, a rather high rate of spontaneous or nonvisually induced dysrhythmia was observed. Eighteen of the thirty-four cases had paroxysmal dysrhythmia, with or without clinical seizures, in the resting, sleep, or sensory-deprived state. This high figure is undoubtedly due to the prolonged periods of time for which the patients were observed in these states and during treatment sessions. While epileptic manifestations other than photosensitivity were also at work in these patients, the invariable occurrences of dysrhythmia with the appropriate stimulus confirmed that these patients also had visually induced epilepsy.

While most patients with photosensitivity do not have obvious structural diseases of the nervous system, the condition has been reported in association with cerebellar degeneration,[21] Alzheimer's disease,[22] cerebral palsy,[23] and subsequent to head injuries.[24]

Two patients in this series had cerebellar degeneration with myoclonic seizures and photosensitivity (Cases 21 and 26). There were two instances of cerebral palsy, one patient had suffered a head injury as noted before, and one patient (Case 3) had a trisomy-D abnormality and numerous congenital anomalies.

Case 38 with multiple sclerosis had photosensitivity, pattern, and eye closure dysrhythmia. The relationship of the evoked dysrhythmia to the underlying disease process was difficult to evaluate. Seizures are known to occur in multiple sclerosis, and so photoconvulsive responses might reasonably be obtained. It should be noted that this was the only patient in the series who did not complain of or have incidences of clinical seizures. She was included to note the occurrence of visually induced dysrhythmia in a case of multiple sclerosis.

Since most of the patients were from distant cities, and the families were not available, no systematic laboratory survey was made of the relatives of the patients in this study. Therefore, no detailed studies of genetic factors were made. However, the high incidence of seizures in the family histories suggests a genetic factor. The family history was positive for seizure disorders in eighteen of the thirty-six families whose family histories were known.

Heredity certainly plays a role in at least some instances, for example, in the family reported by Schwartz.[25] In his family, the father and all four children were photosensitive while the mother's responses were normal. The observations which were made during this study tend to support this concept, especially the occurrence of photosensitivity in Cases 7 and 8 who are brothers. Their age of onset and frequency characteristics were identical, and their IQs were similar; 95 and 97. Daly and Bickford[26] reported the occurrence of photosensitivity in identical twins while Tan[27] reported it in only one case involving identical twins.

Most of the patients in the study had by history both major and minor seizures, the major seizures being convulsions or generalized major motor attacks. The minor seizures were also generalized and were petit mal types of attacks, "absence" in character but frequently accompanied by myoclonic jerking movements.

The intellectual levels of the patients varied considerably. One patient was a college graduate. From the data listed in Table II it is impossible to draw a conclusion associating photosensitivity with intellectual development. That photosensitivity can occur with serious impairment is obvious, as for example in

Case 3, the unfortunate youngster with trisomy-D abnormality.

The pathophysiological mechanisms are not known for photosensitive epilepsy. The EEG dysrhythmia is predominantly wave and spike in type but often atypical. With the bilateral wave and spike dysrhythmia present, the reticular formation is naturally assumed to play at least some role in the process. But in some instances, the dysrhythmia had been localized to the posterior region of the hemispheres. This led to the premise that two factors are necessary for the evocation; (a) the arrival of afferent stimuli to (b) a cortical area exhibiting hyperexcitability.[10]

Patients with photic-induced epilepsy are known to be less sensitive to flickering light when asleep.[28, 29] Rodin, Daly, and Bickford[30] studied normal subjects and photosensitive patients, awake and asleep, and found by low frequency analysis in normal subjects that driving of the cortex occurs with photic stimulation but is less marked when asleep. The difference in responses obtained in the waking and sleeping states is largely one of degree. The driving occurs in photosensitive patients, but the photoconvulsive effect is less marked both clinically and electroencephalographically during sleep. This indicates an elevated threshold. However, the normal driving of the cortex occurs. Rodin, Daly, and Bickford postulated a "leakage" from the optic system which activates the spike-wave center, and they assumed the leakage occurs between the lateral geniculate body and the epileptic focus.

PATTERN-EVOKED EPILEPSY

Bickford[16] reported the first case of pattern-evoked epilepsy. Subsequent cases have been reported by Bickford and Klass,[17] Gastaut and Tassinari,[31] Chatrian,[32, 33] and Forster.[34] The case previously reported by the author is Case 37 in the series of cases of visually induced epilepsy.

Fourteen of the patients studied had seizures or dysrhythmia evoked by the viewing of patterns. Ten of these fourteen patients were also photosensitive, and one of the remaining four also had dysrhythmia evoked by eye closure. Three patients had pattern epilepsy only.

In two of the ten patients with both pattern-evoked epilepsy and photosensitivity, the pattern sensitivity was of greater clinical importance than was the photosensitivity (Cases 25 and 27).

The seizures in all patients were of the minor absence type and the accompanying dysrhythmia was of the atypical generalized wave and spike type. The duration and severity of the evoked dysrhythmia varied even in the same patient upon repeated presentations (Figs. 7A and 7B).

These patients were predominantly female (12:2) and varied in age from two to twenty-four years. The two-year-old appeared to be retarded and certainly was slow in reaching milestones of development; one patient aged thirteen years was definitely retarded, but the others were of normal intelligence, and indeed, one was a college graduate.

The patterns which evoked dysrhythmia were the horizontal and vertical black lines on white paper, screen grids, and a pattern with radiating lines (a "sunburst" type of pattern). Also employed were some three-dimensional patterns, but these were not effective in evoking dysrhythmias. Upon the request of the author, the families photographed particular views which had attracted the patients and where they had self-induced their seizures. These included the picture of a wall of a school building (Case 27). The wall was frame, and with the customary shingling effect, the overlap of the boards resembled the line drawings. In another patient, viewing a brick fireplace in her home evoked seizures (Case 34).

All fourteen of the study patients with significant pattern-induced epilepsy were monocularly insensitive, a point also discussed by Chatrian.[32, 33] Chatrian points out as well the importance of the angle of viewing and the role of straight lines.

EYE CLOSURE DYSRHYTHMIA

Upon eye closure, significant dysrhythmia ocurred in four of the patients in this series (Fig. 8). A fifth, prior case was published[34] with eye closure dysrhythmia and without photosensitivity. A breakdown of the figures according to sex shows three females and two males. In the four patients in this series, as with the prior case, patching of one eye precluded the appearance of the dysrhythmia, when the nonpatched eye was closed

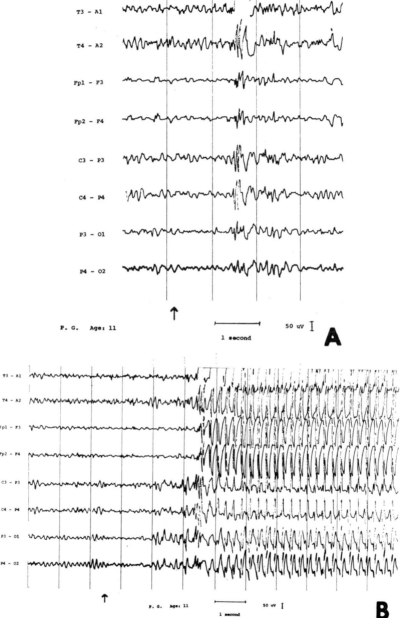

Figure 7. Pattern epilepsy. Arrows indicate points of eye opening with viewing of patterns. 7A shows short burst of multiple spikes and atypical slow wave evoked by horizontal lines. 7B shows prolonged burst of atypical spike-wave dysrhythmia generalized but beginning occipitally. Both dysrhythmias evoked by viewing radiating lines. Case 25.

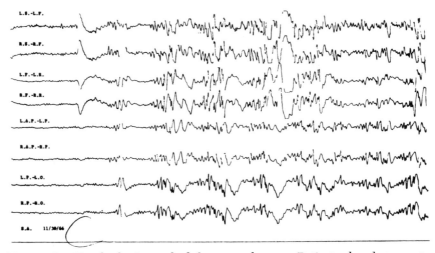

Figure 8.   Dysrhythmia evoked by eye closure. Patient closed eyes at point where technician wrote "C." Top four channels show simultaneously eye blink artifact. Marked dysrrhythmia begins one second later. Illumination in laboratory 600 footcandles. Reprinted from *Cond Reflex*, 2:236, 1967.

in the presence of a bright light. Also, in all five patients, when the room was darkened and the patient closed his/her eyes, no dysrhythmia occurred (Fig. 9). This demonstrates that eye-closure dysrhythmia or epilepsy is a visually induced epilepsy and is not due to proprioceptive feedback from the eye lids. If the proprioceptive feedback was a factor, the dysrhythmia would be present when the eyes are closed in the dark. Moreover, the darkness itself cannot be the evoking factor. The case reported by Giovanardi et al.,[35] however, demonstrates a different mechanism. In Giovanardi's patient, either closing the eyes or darkening the room would produce seizures, and opening the eyes or turning on the light inhibited the attacks.

OBJECT/COLOR-EVOKED EPILEPSY

Seizures elicited by the observance of a particular object are extremely rare. Klass and Daly[36] reported a child who had such seizures upon viewing his left hand. The evoking object need not be a body part; for example, in the patient of Mitchell,

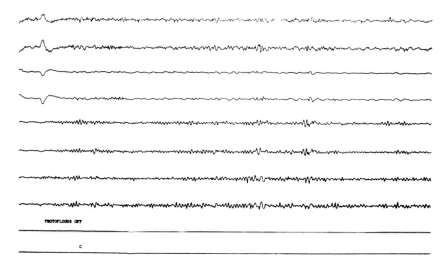

PHOTOFLOODS OFF

c

Figure 9. Same patient. Eye closure in darkened room. Eye blink artifact present in top four channels. No dysrhythmia evoked. Reprinted from
Cond Reflex, 2:236, 1967.

Falconer, and Hill[37] the viewing of a safety pin evoked seizures.

While there are references to the role of various colors in
photosensitivity, there are only two references in the literature
to the induction of seizures by the presentation of a specific color.
The first is that of Kojima et al.,[38] of a seven-year-old boy who
had seizures while watching television. This was found to be
related not to flicker but rather due to the presentation of red
light; in the laboratory, placing the child in a red light evoked
wave and spike dysrhythmia. The second report[18] is an abstract
of a patient in the study (Case 39) who had seizures upon
viewing the color red or viewing an object—his hand. Because
of the rarity of these conditions, he is reported in some detail.

CASE 39. This patient, a five-year-old white male, was the
product of an unremarkable pregnancy and delivery but was
noted to have jerking movements of his arms at the age of five
months. An EEG at the age of seven months was reported as
showing "hypsarhythmia." He walked at the age of twenty
months but never developed speech.

At the age of two years he began inducing seizures, usually
in a series. The first seizure induced in a series was tonic in

type. The subsequent evoked seizures were myoclonic jerks. He induced these seizures by seeking out red objects and hunching over them until a seizure occurred. If he was in a room with a shelf of books, he would remove one with a red binding, carry it to a chair or place it on the floor, and hunch over it. If he found a magazine, he would leaf through it until a bright red object appeared, and he would again do the same. In a group of people, he would seek out those wearing red clothing. For example, at a picnic he followed a young lady in plaid slacks, stood directly behind her, staring at a red part of the plaid until he fell. Shortly after recovery from the tonic seizure, he arose, sought out the young lady, stared again at the red patch and induced a series of myoclonic seizures.

When red objects were not available, he could induce seizures by hunching over his hand and moving the digits; the same sequence of seizures could then be evoked.

The family history was negative for central nervous system disease. The patient was the third child in a family of five children with ages ranging from two to ten years.

The past medical history revealed the patient was jaundiced a few days after birth, but this cleared spontaneously. He had received measles vaccine. Toilet training was the limit of his training capacity.

On physical examination, no congenital deformities were found and the body and face were symmetrical. He did not interact with people and had no speech, though he did utter sounds. The physical examination was otherwise normal.

During neurological examination he did not respond to the examiner. He was uncooperative. During the course of the examination he continuously attempted to induce seizures. His attention span was short, except when he was inducing seizures. His cranial nerves were grossly intact. Motor examination revealed that muscle tone was normal, and he used all extremities equally. The strength of all the extremities and the trunk muscles was within normal limits. The deep tendon reflexes were hypoactive but symmetrical, and there were no pathological reflexes.

The sensory examination was difficult to evaluate, but the patient withdrew to pinprick on all extremities. Cerebellar tests and coordination tests were grossly normal in the upper and lower extremities, but the gait tended to be wide-based most of the time. He often walked on his toes but was also able to walk with a normal gait.

In the laboratory, the mother's account of the seizures was verified. When placed in a crib with a number of toys he quickly sought out one with prominent red markings, hunched over it and induced seizures (Fig. 10). Also, when the toys were removed and a magazine placed in his crib he quickly leafed through it to find advertisements with red coloring and began the process. When left alone in the crib without red objects or pictures, he hunched over, staring at his hand, moved his digits, and induced seizures (Fig. 11).

Usually the first seizure was a tonic seizure with extension of all extremities lasting five to six seconds, with suppression of

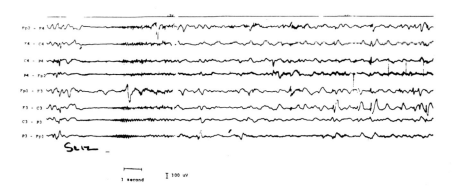

Figure 10. Color-induced epilepsy. Patient hunched over a red object. and stiffened in a short tonic seizure ("Seiz"). This began at the point in the EEG tracing when the flattening of the record occurred. The low voltage fast activity was followed by spiking discharges especially in the F3-C3 recording. Case 39.

brain activity followed by focal spiking discharges. This is similar to the dysrhythmia described by Klass and Daly[36] in object-evoked epilepsy.

Subsequent seizures were myoclonic in type with spiking discharges, and the seizures gradually decreased in severity. When he finally was unable to evoke a seizure from a red object, he would relinquish it, only to return to it or another red object after five or ten minutes and, if the extinction phase was over, would then begin the process again.

When red objects were not available and he induced seizures by viewing his left hand, the same sequence of seizures and EEG changes occurred. The seizures evoked by viewing either red objects or his hand were monocularly induced with either

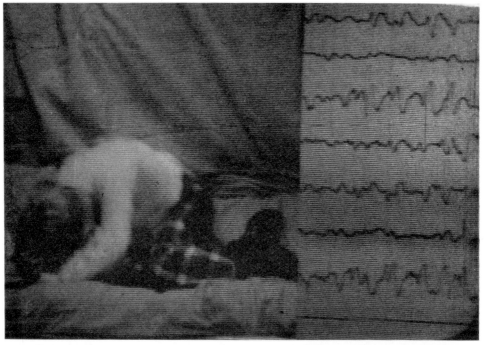

Figure 11.   Same patient. Seizures evoked by looking at object; his hand. Myoclonic seizure. Note elevation of left leg. EEG shows spiking dysrhythmia most prominent in occipital leads (channels three and seven from the top).

eye. The seizures did not occur immediately but required from several seconds to minutes of stimulation for induction.

When the lighting in the EEG laboratory was altered to a red lamp, the spontaneously occurring dysrhythmia was markedly increased. Also when the patient was asleep, changing the room light to red increased the paroxysmal dysrhythmia.

SELF-INDUCTION OF VISUALLY INDUCED SEIZURES

The phenomenon of patients inducing their own seizures is usually considered a peculiarity of the visually induced types of seizures. It may occur in other forms however. As discussed in Chapter 7, one of the study patients with somatosensory-evoked epilepsy induced attacks in order to control his seizures. He could, after the induction of a seizure in the morning, proceed safely about his business for the rest of the day. Here the self-induction was employed for preventive therapy. In musicogenic epilepsy self-induction, or attempts at it, may serve a secondary gain as described in Chapter 15. By and large however, self-induction is most common in the visually induced epilepsies.

Many photoconvulsive patients can evoke their seizures by rapid eye blinking or, more commonly, by finger waving. The latter is accomplished by looking at a bright light and rapidly passing the spread fingers back and forth before the eyes thus producing an intermittent stimulation.

This is said to be uncommon, and Andermann et al.[39] pooling the data from nine clinics in different countries found thirty-four cases, twenty-one of whom were definitely shown to be self-inducers. In the University of Wisconsin study series of photo-sensitive patients, nine were known to have self-induced seizures by finger waving. One of these patients had a convulsion in 1969 and in the course of the workup was found to be photo-sensitive. The family, on reviewing home movies of the Christmas of 1967—two years before she was known to have seizures—noted the hand waving and drop attack. In the laboratory in 1969 a seizure was elicited by hand-waving (*see* Fig. 6).

One of the ten patients with both photosensitivity and pattern epilepsy (Case 27) induced attacks only by pattern evocation and never by finger-waving. She would stand and stare at a particular wall at her school which was characterized by distinct horizontal lines. Three of the four patients with only pattern epilepsy also induced their attacks. Case 34, a retarded two-year-old, spent much of her time at home staring at the design of the brick fireplace in the family living room, thus inducing seizures. As noted above, self-stimulation was a prominent part of the picture in the child with color/object-induced epilepsy.

The reason these patients self-stimulate is not clear, despite the abundant literature on this matter.[39-46] Self-stimulation has been related to mental retardation, but this is certainly not true in all patients. Several of our self-inducing patients were superior high school students. They have in general been unable to tell why they do this although occasionally a patient, as occurred in two cases in the study, will resort to this device to avoid household chores.

There have been some suggestions of autoeroticism and a likening to masturbation as explanatory constructs. This may be true in a few instances, but there is no persuasive reason to believe it applies to the majority. In regard to erotic components, however, the case observed by Ehret et al.[19] for thirty-two years induced attacks which were followed by sexual stimulation, even to the point of criminal offense.

Also, during emotional stresses, patients may use this device as a retreat from unpleasant situations. It has been described as a habit tic spasm.[41] Some have felt it is part of the seizure itself,[45] but one would doubt this since it can be reproduced on command in the laboratory. In one patient (Case 30) it was noted that self-induction occurred when she was bored or upset.

This chapter presents the study of thirty-nine patients with visually induced epilepsy and compares them with the cases reported in the literature. While the visually induced forms of epilepsy are the most common of the reflex epilepsies, rare forms exist within this category.

The detailed methods of studying the individual patient have been presented. The importance of searching for more than one type of visually induced epilepsy in the same patient is stressed.

The factors determined by the careful study are thus outlined: monocular insensitivity, degree of sensitivity with eyes open and closed, exact frequency ranges, and intensity of stimulus are important for the determination of behavioral treatment.

REFERENCES

1. Celesia, G. C.: Personal communication (paper to be submitted).
2. Lennox, W. G.: *Epilepsy and related disorders.* Boston, Little, *1*:365, 1960.
3. Gowers, W.: *Epilepsy and Other Chronic Convulsive Disorders.* New York, Wm. Wood, 1885.
4. Ranney, A.: *Nervous Disease.* Philadelphia, Davis, 1882.
5. Holmes, G.: Local epilepsy. *Lancet, 1*:957, 1927.
6. Cobb, S.: Photic driving as a cause of clinical seizures in epileptic patients. *Arch Neurol Psychiat, 58*:70, 1947.
7. Gastaut, H., Roger, J., and Gastaut, Y.: Experimental forms of human epilepsy. Epilepsy induced by rhythmic intermittent luminous stimulation (photogenic epilepsy). *Rev Neurol, 80*:161, 1948.
8. Gastaut, H.: L'Epilepsie photgenique. *Rev Prat, 1*:105, 1951.
9. Bickford, R. G., Daly, D., and Keith, H. M.: Convulsive effects of light stimulation in children. *Amer J Dis Child, 86*:170, 1953.
10. Gangelberger, J. A. and Cvetko, B.: Photogene epilepsie, *Wien Z Nervenheilkd, 13*:22, 1956.
11. Naquet, R., Fergersten, L., and Bert, J.: Seizure discharges localized to the posterior cerebral regions in man provoked by intermittent photic stimulation. *Electroencephalogr Clin Neurophysiol, 12*:305, 1960.
12. Pazzaglia, P., Sabattini, L., and Lugaresi, E.: Crisi occipitali precipitate dal buio. *Rev Neurol, 40*:184, 1970.
13. Forster, F. M. and Campos, G. B.: Conditioning factors in stroboscopic-induced seizures. *Epilepsia, 5*:156, 1964.
14. Forster, F. M., Ptacek, L. J., Peterson, W. G., and Chun, R. W. M.: Stroboscopic-induced seizures altered by extinction techniques. *Trans Am Neurol Assoc, 89*:136, 1964.
15. Marshall, C., Walker, A. E., and Livingston, S.: Photogenic epilepsy; parameters of activation. *Arch Neurol Psychiat, 69*:760, 1953.
16. Bickford, R. G. and Klass, D. W.: Stimulus factors in the mechanism of television-induced seizures. *Trans Am Neurol Assoc, 87*:176, 1962.
17. Bickford, R. G. and Klass, D. W.: Trigger mechanisms in visual pattern epilepsy. Symposium on Basic Mechanisms of the Epilepsies, Colorado Springs, Colorado, November, 1968.

18. Forster, F. M.: Seizures, induced by viewing specific color or object. *Trans Am Neurol Assoc, 97*:284, 1972.
19. Doose, H., Giesler, K., and Volzke, E.: Observations in photosensitive children with and without epilepsy. *Z Kinderheilkd, 107*:26, 1969.
20. Ehert, R. and Schneider, E.: Photogenic epilepsy with habitual self-provoked petit mal attacks and repeated sex offense. *Arch Psychiat Nervenkr, 202*:75, 1961.
21. Lamartine de Assis, J., Freitas Julio, A., and Russo, G.: Epilepsia mioclónica. Estudio clínico electroencephalográphico. *Arch Neuro Psychiat, 51*:215, 1957.
22. Gimenez, R., Peraita, S., Lopez, P., and Agreda, J. M. et al.: Myoclonus and photic induced seizures in Alzheimer's disease. *Eur Neurol, 5*:215, 1971.
23. Daly, D. D., Siekert, R. G., and Burke, E. C.: A variety of familial light sensitive epilepsy. *Electroencephalogr Clin Neurophysiol, 11*:141, 1959.
24. Neugebauer, W.: Uber photostimulation effekt un Unfall bei Hirnverletzten. *Dtsch Z Ges Gerichtl Med, 49*:644, 1960.
25. Davidson, S. and Watson, C. W.: Hereditary light sensitive epilepsy. *Neurology, 6*:233, 1956.
26. Daly, D. and Bickford, R. G.: Electroencephalographic studies of identical twins with photo-epilepsy. *Electroencephalogr Clin Neurophysiol, 3*:245, 1956.
27. Tan, M.: A case of photogenic epilepsy in an identical twin. *Psychiat Neurol Jap, 65*:184, 1963.
28. Scollo-Lavizzari, G. and Hess, R.: Photic stimulation during paradoxical sleep in photosensitive patients. *Neurology, 17*:604, 1967.
29. Yamamoto, J., Furuya, E., Wakamatsu, H., and Hishikawa, Y.: Modification of photosensitivity in epileptics during sleep. *Electroencephalogr Clin Neurophysiol, 31*:509, 1971.
30. Rodin, E. A., Daly, D. D., and Bickford, R. G.: Effects of photic stimulation during sleep. *Neurology, 5*:149, 1955.
31. Gastaut, H. and Tassinari, C. A.: Triggering mechanisms in epilepsy. The electrical point of view. *Epilepsia, 7*:85, 1966.
32. Chatrian, G. E., Lettich, E., Miller, L. H., and Green, J. R.: Pattern-sensitive epilepsy. Part 1. An electrographic study of its mechanisms. *Epilepsia, 11*:125, 1970.
33. Chatrian, G. E., Lettich, E., Miller, L. H., Green, J. R., and Kupfer, C.: Pattern-sensitive epilepsy, Part 2. Clinical changes, tests of responsiveness and motor output, alterations of evoked potentials and therapeutic measures. *Epilepsia, 11*:151, 1970.
34. Forster, F. M.: Conditioning of cerebral dysrhythmia induced by pattern presentation and eye closure. *Cond Reflex, 2*:236, 1967.
35. Giovanardi Rossi, P., Frank, L., and Pazzaglia, P.: Crisi epilettiche alla chiusura degli occi. *G Psichiat Neuropat, 97*:467, 1969.

36. Klass, D. and Daly, D. D.: An unusual seizure induction mechanism ("manugenic"). *Electroencephalogr Clin Neurophysiol, 12:*756, 1960.
37. Mitchell, W., Falconer, M. A., and Hill, D.: *Lancet, 2:*626, 1954.
38. Kojima, K., Suguro, T., Miyamoto, K., Inazumi, H., and Sakaya, S.: Photogenic epilepsy. Television aspect. *J Pediat Proct* (Tokyo), *26:*1377, 1963.
39. Anderman, K. et al.: Self-induced epilepsy. *Arch Neurol, 6:*49, 1962.
40. Green, J. B.: Self-induced seizure. *Arch Neurol, 15:*579, 1966.
41. Robertson, E. G.: Photogenic epilepsy. Self-induced attacks. *Brain,* 77:232, 1956.
42. Hutchinson, J. H., Stone, F. H., and Davidson, J. R.: Photogenic epilepsy induced by the patient. *Lancet, 1:*243, 1958.
43. Kammerer, T.: Suchtiges Verhalten bei Epilepsia, Photogene Epilepsie mit selbstinduzierten Anfallen. *Dsch Z Nervenheilk, 185:*319, 1963.
44. Harley, R. D., Baird, H. W., and Freeman, R. D.: Self-induced photogenic epilepsy. *Arch Ophthalmol,* 78:730, 1967.
45. Ames, F. R.: Self-induction in photosensitive epilepsy. *Brain, 94:*781, 1971.
46. Clement, C. P., Andermann, F., and Dongier, F. I.: Self-induced epilepsy, a study of two patients. *Epilepsia, 16:*202, 1975.

CHAPTER 3

EPILEPSY EVOKED BY AUDITORY STIMULI

AUDITORY-EVOKED EPILEPSY was first described by Gowers[1] at the turn of the century, and there are numerous subsequent reports by others.[2-16] The earliest reported cases were those referred to as startle or acousticomotor epilepsy and were precipitated by the sudden, loud, unexpected presentation of a sound stimulus. It should be noted, however, that the term "startle" also includes cases with seizures evoked by modalities other than auditory. This occurs, for example, in some cases of somatosensory epilepsy. Therefore, the term "startle" does not necessarily mean auditory-evoked. Moreover, there are also other forms of auditory-evoked epilepsy, as noted below.

In the group of patients with seizures evoked by auditory stimuli, there are variations in (a) the nature of the sound stimulus, (b) whether or not a surprise or startling factor is necessary, and (c) the type of seizure evoked by the stimulus.

The nature of the sound stimulus may vary. In many patients any sudden, loud, nonspecific noise as the dropping of a dish, backfiring of an engine, breaking of glass, or a shot will induce a seizure. In other patients, the sound needs to be very discrete and specific, such as a telephone bell or a particular voice.

The surprise element plays a prominent role in some patients. Generally the element of surprise is necessary for the evocation of seizures in those patients whose seizures are evoked by a nonspecific loud noise, although there are exceptions to this as noted below.

In the literature, various types of seizures have been described as being evoked by sounds. These include:

1. Myoclonic-absences; Cohen et al.,[7] Strobos,[8] Gastaut et al.,[9, 10] Booker and Forster[11]

44

2. Tonic seizures; Strobos[8]
3. Psychomotor automatisms; Peet, Daly, and Bickford[12]
4. Adversive seizures; Peet, Daly, and Bickford[12]
5. Adversive seizures progressing to a major motor; Foerster[13] and Forster[14]
6. Focal, aphasic; Forster et al.[15]

In addition to the above, there are the tonic or sometimes clonic movements occurring without significant EEG component in patients with hemiparesis.[16] Critchley[3] feels that the latter are probably exaggerated acousticomotor reflexes in children with spastic paresis and that any sudden loud noise often exaggerates myoclonic or tonic reactions, particularly in the paretic limbs and probably on the basis of lack of proper inhibition.

The University of Wisconsin study included fifteen instances of auditory-evoked epilepsy. Table IV presents the number of cases, the nature of the auditory stimulus, whether a startling component was necessary, and the type of seizures evoked.

Short descriptions of these patients (except for the musico-genic patients) follow under the appropriate headings used in Table IV.

TABLE IV

PATIENTS WITH AUDITORY-EVOKED EPILEPSY

	Type of Auditory Stimulus	*Startling or Nonstartling*	*Types of Seizures*	*Case Number*
A.	Nonspecific noise	Startle	Myoclonic	1, 2, 3
B.	Nonspecific noise	Startle	Tonic	4, 5
C.	Nonspecific noise	Startle	Focal motor to major motor	6
D.	Specific (telephone)	Startle	Psychomtor	7
E.	Specific (telephone)	Nonstartle	Major motor	8
F.	Nonspecific voices	Startle	Major motor	9
G.	Specific voices	Nonstartle	Major motor and aphasic to focal	10
	Specific music	Nonstartle	Psychomotor	1-5 (Chap. 4)

A. Acousticomotor or Startle Epilepsy Evoked by Sudden Unexpected Nonspecific Noise

Cases 1, 2, and 3 are examples of myoclonic-absence types of seizures evoked by nonspecific noises. These patients had seizures evoked in the laboratory upon presentation of any startling noise, provided it was loud enough, was unexpected, and was presented binaurally. The kinds of noises presented were gun shots, sonic booms, sound of dropping utensils, and various alarm bells and buzzers. These sounds were recorded on audiotape, and the presentations were randomized, i.e. the time between presentations varied from a few seconds to five minutes (with and wtihout distracting stimuli). The distracting stimuli consisted of music, engaging the patient in conversation, and projection of appropriate slides of travelogs. The presentations were either free field or through special stereo earphones which permitted either binaural or (by eliminating the stimulus to either ear) monaural presentations. When the sounds were presented monaurally, no seizure occurred, provided the sound level was below 60 decibels. Sounds louder than this become binaural due to bone conduction. Cases 1 and 2 have been reported previously.[11]

CASE 1. This patient, a ten-year-old male, suffered from frequent myoclonic seizures in response to sudden sounds. The attacks involved the upper extremities and, to a lesser extent, the head and neck. Mild jaundice on the fourth day of life was accompanied by a generalized seizure. Three generalized seizures occurred during the next three weeks, but there were no recurrences of these after the first four weeks of life. At age sixteen months, an evaluation for delayed motor development suggested cerebral palsy, and a pneumoencephalogram at that time showed cortical atrophy. At eight years, focal clonic attacks of the left arm and left leg occurred. They could be avoided occasionally by the patient holding the left wrist firmly with his right hand. At about this same time, generalized myoclonic or startle responses to sound began to occur. At the time of evaluation, the patient walked with crutches and showed a marked spastic paraparesis. Routine electroencephalogram revealed a nonspecific dysrhythmia.

CASE 2. This patient, a thirteen-year-old male, suffered from persistent myoclonic startle responses to sound, involving primarily the upper extremities but also the facial musculature, with extension of the neck and spine. Any sudden noise would evoke a brief startle seizure. He was severely retarded, secondary to anoxia at birth. The myoclonic attacks were first noted at age nine months. A pneumoencephalogram at ten months showed diffuse cortical atrophy. At the time of study, he was severely retarded with flexion deformities of all extremities. His routine electroencephalogram showed a marked, nonspecific dysrhythmia.

CASE 3. This patient has not been previously reported. This two-year-old white male had had, from the age of fifteen months, abnormal responses to unexpected noises and, to some extent, to tactile stimulation. When startled by noise, his eyes rolled up, there were several generalized myoclonic jerks, and the patient was temporarily unresponsive. These episodes lasted up to ten seconds; the patient then appeared entirely normal. The child often dropped objects during these episodes, and the episodes occurred as often as twenty-five to forty times a day. There had been no major motor or other seizures.

There was no history of head trauma or high and prolonged fever. The patient was the product of a normal pregnancy, but the mother felt that she was oversedated at the time of delivery, and the baby was sleepy for some time postpartum.

The patient was previously studied elsewhere, and was found on several occasions to have right temporal spiking and slow waves on the EEG. On one occasion, some frontal slow waves were noted as well.

The patient had been treated with phenobarbital, diphenyl-hydantoin, diazepam, and amphetamines, with no significant change in seizure pattern.

Review of systems was noncontributory, and there was a history of diabetes and pernicious anemia on the maternal side of the family.

On physical examination, the patient was an alert, cooperative, well-developed, and well-nourished child. He was somewhat hyperactive. The patient had four to five startle episodes during the examination. The child spoke only in short phrases and did not use sentences. His head was normocephalic. Neurological examination was normal except for the induced attacks.

Laboratory and X-ray studies, including skull films, were normal. Sabin dye test was negative for toxoplasmosis.

RESEARCH STUDIES

These three patients when studied in the Research Laboratory were all found to have seizures reliably evoked by sudden, unexpected, loud noises of various types, upon random presentations as noted above. The electroencephalograms during the induced attacks in Cases 1 and 2 were difficult to interpret (Fig. 12), and it was not certain that they did not represent movement artifact rather than cortical electrical disturbance.

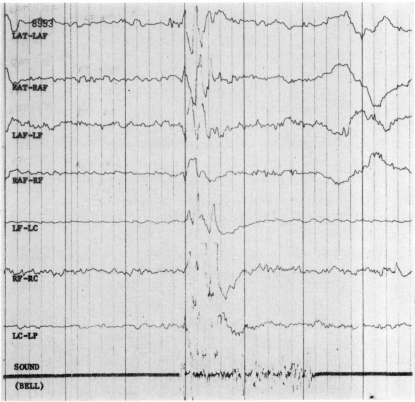

Figure 12.   EEG tracing in Case 1, Chapter 3. Bottom channel is sound indicator and indicates the presentation of the sound stimulus. The changes noted in the EEG were due to movement artifact, as they did not occur when the stimulus was administered after the patient had received Anectine®. Reprinted from *Neurology* © 1965 by The New York Times Media Company, Inc.

The administration of Anectine prior to the delivery of the stimulus showed no abnormality in the EEG when the myoclonic movement was thus pervented.[11] From this it was deduced that the changes recorded in the EEG were essentially movement artifact, and the seizures were subcortical and in accordance with the description of Critchley.[3] The changes in EEG recordings were probably akin to that seen in photomyoclonus. In the third case, however, the elicited EEG was of the spike-wave complex type, generalized and persisting upon termination of the stimulus. This was definitely a centrencephalic type of dysrhythmia (Fig. 13), probably of secondary type. These cases therefore include both subcortical and cortical kinds of acousticomotor epilepsy.

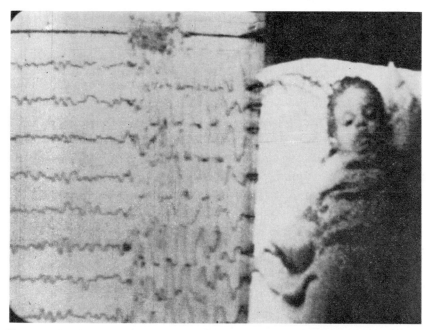

Figure 13. From AV tape recording. Case 3, Chapter 3. Patient in myoclonic seizure evoked by sudden noise. Left arm jerking upwards. Top channel of EEG is a noise indicator, showing the time of presentation of· the sound stimulus—a buzzer. Sound evoked atypical spike-slow wave dysrhythmia. Reprinted from *Physiological Effects of Noise*, Plenum Press, 1970.

B.   *Tonic Seizures Evoked by Unexpected Nonspecific Noises*

Tonic seizures may represent an exaggerated acousticomotor reflex and not really be epileptic as pointed out by Critchley,[3] Wabayashi et al.,[5] Strobos,[8] and in Case 4 cited herein. However, as in Case 5, the attacks may be definitely cerebral and epileptic in nature.

While the tonic component is most prominent in these seizures, there may be unilateral clonic movements. Frequently these patients are severely brain damaged, have hemiparesis with spasticity and may also have smallness of the involved body parts. The following case is an example of this type of acousticomotor response.

CASE 4.   This patient was an eighteen-year-old girl with the chief complaint of shaking of her left arm and leg. She was healthy until the age of seven months when she had meningitis, secondary to a right otitis media. The meningitis was treated with penicillin and sulfadiazine. At the age of eight months, the parents noted shaking episodes in her left arm. These continued episodically, and were described as being shiverlike, of high frequency and of low amplitude movements, and as occurring with a definite relationship to startle and sound. They were not associated with any pains, paresthesias or aura. Since the age of sixteen years, the involuntary movements of the left arm were associated with similar involuntary movements of the left leg. None of the standard anticonvulsant medications alleviated the seizures.

Physical examination was normal. The neurological examination revealed slightly more difficulty in standing on the left leg than on the right, and slight circumduction of the left leg occurred when walking. There was smallness of body parts on the left, with about 2 cm difference in hand width. Motor power and tone were normal in the right upper extremity. There was slight spasticity at the left elbow and moderate at the left wrist and left fingers. Hand patting movements were decreased. There was a moderate increase in deep tendon reflexes in the left upper extremity along with a slight difficulty with posture in the left lower extremity. The plantar signs were normal on the right and suggestive on the left. Vibration, position, pinprick, and pinprick localization were normal throughout, but there was some difficulty in stereognosis in the left hand, while texture discrimination was normal. Weight discrimination was decreased on both sides, but graphesthesia was normal.

The laboratory studies were within normal limits except for the following: The neuropsychological testing data was indicative of right hemisphere impairment. The routine awake EEG showed a dysrhythmia, grade II in type and generalized. Sleep EEG activated focal spikes in the right frontal area which became generalized.

When studied in the Research Laboratory it was obvious that she had sound-induced seizures. However, the evoked seizures were not accompanied by significant electroencephalographic changes.

Considerable muscle artifact was present in the recordings, but a definitive and epileptogenic change could not be discerned. This patient is therefore similar to those described by Critchley.[3]

Her seizures were induced by sudden loud noises of varying types, e.g. rifle shot, buzzer, bell, and the sound of dropping metallic objects. They could also be induced by skin shocks administered over either the left or right side of the body and by other somatosensory stimuli, such as removing the masking tape that was holding the shock electrodes. She herself was aware of occasionally having seizures when she bumped into objects. The somatosensory-evoked component was less obvious to her, and indeed, except for those induced by electric shock, the seizures were not nearly as constant as were the auditory-induced seizures. The seizures were tonic, occasionally with some clonic component of the left arm and leg and, at times, of the left face.

Tonic seizures evoked by sudden, nonspecific, and unexpected sounds may, however, be truly epileptic, as was the case in the next patient described. His tonic seizures were accompanied by a significant EEG dysrhythmia.

CASE 5. This patient, a sixteen-year-old male high school student, was first in birth order, and his birth was prolonged and traumatic. He was noted early to have motor impairment on the right side. At the age of about six years, he began having episodes of stiffness and elevation of the right arm. These were evoked by noises of varying types, but only if the sound was unexpected. Sometimes the click of a spoon against a plate, sometimes the sound of his father's or mother's voice (especially when giving sharp commands), and, at other times, the dropping of a dish evoked the movement. They apparently also were known to occur spontaneously.

In some episodes, instead of the localized phenomenon in the right arm, he "stiffened like a board and fell backward." Adequate anticonvulsant medication did not control the seizures.

Neurological examination was normal except for the following: There was a very slight right lower facial weakness on both voluntary and mimetic movement. There was obvious smallness of the length and breadth of the right hand and right foot, and the right leg was slightly shorter. The nipple to midsternal line distance was decreased by 2 cm on the right, and the scapula was obviously smaller on the right than on the left. The smallness of body parts was associated with a very slight increase in muscle tone, especially at the finger joints. There was marked digital weakness in the right upper and lower extremities. There was slight intention tremor on finger-to-nose test, with rebound phenomenon and dyssynergia on toe-to-object test in the right extremities. The deep tendon reflexes were increased on the right side and were accompanied by a Hoffmann's sign. The plantar signs were normal bilaterally. Vibratory, position, pin-prick, and pinprick localization sensations were all normal, but two-point discrimination was markedly decreased in the right upper extremity.

When studied in the Research Laboratory, EEGs in the rest-ing, sleep and sensory-deprived state were normal. When, how-ever, a sudden, unexpected auditory stimulus was administered, the tonic seizures occurred and were accompanied by an evoked EEG dysrhythmia (Fig. 14). This response was consistently obtained when startling sounds were administered. There was no specificity to the type of auditory stimulus.

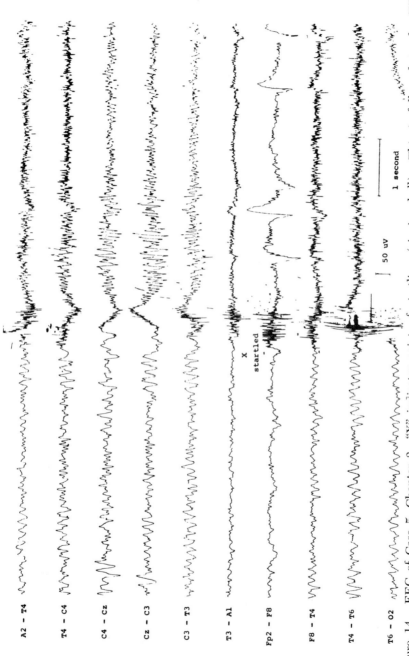

Figure 14. EEG of Case 5, Chapter 3. "X" indicates point of startling (ringing bell). This is followed in the EEG tracings by movement artifact, then muscle artifact. Fast spiking discharges followed, most prominent from electrode Cz. During this time patient's right arm was in a tonic seizure.

C.   Focal to Major Motor Seizures Induced by Startling, Nonspecific Sound

Seizures originating in the temporal lobe may have head-eye deviation as a prominent part of the clinical picture. Peet, Daly and Bickford[12] reported such a patient. The head-eye deviation may proceed to a major motor and generalized seizure as reported by Foerster,[13] and also by Forster.[14] This latter case is again reported here briefly.

CASE 6.   This patient was studied at Jefferson Hospital in 1948, when he was six years old. He was the result of a prolonged and difficult labor, was markedly retarded, and had a marked right hemiparesis with spasticity and smallness of body parts. The retardation was so marked that he had no ability to verbalize, did not respond to his own name, and spent his time using his left hand to spin objects in small circles. Since infancy, he had experienced major motor seizures. While these occurred spontaneously, they were also readily induced by any sudden, loud, unexpected noise. His mother stated that if she dropped a pan in the kitchen and he did not see it in the process of falling, he would have a seizure. If someone unexpectedly knocked on the door or rang the doorbell, a seizure occurred.

X-ray examination of the head revealed marked asymmetry with smallness of the left side of the cranial cavity and thickness of the calvarium on that side. Pneumoencephalogram showed marked dilatation of the left lateral ventricle.

In the laboratory, while he was sitting spinning an ashtray on the floor, an emesis basin was dropped behind him. There was movement artifact and muscle artifact in the EEG, followed by spiking discharges in the left anterior temporal lead. At this point, he had head and eye deviation to the right. The dysrhythmia spread and became generalized, and a major motor seizure ensued with bilateral tonic and clonic movements, loss of consciousness, and postseizure stupor. The EEG in an evoked seizure (Fig. 15) showed a left temporal onset of dysrhythmia.

D.   Seizures Evoked by Specific and Startling Sounds

Up to this point, the patients described in this chapter have had their seizures evoked by nonspecific startling sounds. However, specific sounds, when presented in a startling fashion, have

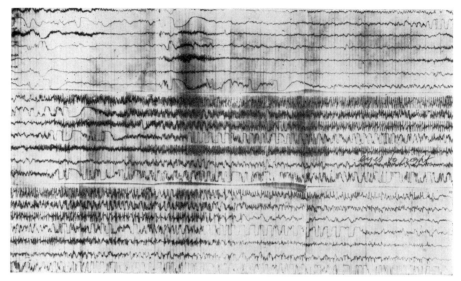

Figure 15. EEG of Case 6, Chapter 3. The stimulus, dropping of a dish behind the patient, evoked movement artifact and muscle artifact followed by spiking dysrhythmia from left temporal electrode (lowest channel) with spread to the other regions, a generalized seizure beginning with deviation to the right. Reprinted from *Arch Medicos de Cuba*, 3:252, 1952.

also been described as evoking seizures. A very precise example is that of Taylor's[17] patient, a soccer player, whose seizures were evoked by the sound of the referee's whistle.

Since psychomotor seizures are a manifestation of temporal lobe epilepsy, and since the auditory cortex is located in the temporal lobe, it is not surprising that acoustic stimulation might evoke psychomotor seizures. This has been reported by Peet, Daly and Bickford.[12] No cases of temporal lobe seizures evoked by nonspecific stimuli were studied in the laboratory, but the following case is an example of a patient who had psychomotor seizures evoked by specific sounds.

CASE 7. This patient, a seventeen-year-old white female, had her first seizure, major motor in type, at the age of fourteen. Subseqently she began having minor seizures. The seizures gradually increased in frequency, unaffected by anticonvulsant medications.

The minor seizures were not preceded by an aura. She first noted shaking of her arms, and they became outstretched and stiff. If she was holding an object, she might either drop it or grasp it tightly, whereupon it could not be taken from her grip. The seizures lasted several minutes and included typical automatisms. There was no history of olfactory, visual, auditory, or Jacksonian seizures. There was no history of trauma, central nervous system infection, or seizures related to fever.

The past and family histories were negative, as were the physical and neurological examination.

Laboratory studies were also normal, including spinal fluid, skull X ray, pneumoencephalogram, and repeated EEGs.

RESEARCH STUDIES

The referring physician commented that this young lady had seizures whenever she was in his office and the telephone rang. Her parents stated that the same happened at home unless she was expecting the phone call. Accordingly, in the laboratory she was exposed to the tapes of startling noises, including loud telephone bells, and no seizure or dysrhythmia was evoked. The telephone instruments used in her county are made by a different manufacturer than the instruments employed in the Madison area. The Iowa County Wisconsin Telephone Company recorded on tape for us the sounds of the instruments in her home and in her doctor's office. When these tapes were played in the laboratory procedure and interspersed with other stimuli, she identified the sound of her telephone instrument, but no seizure occurred. She was constantly on the alert in the laboratory for the presentation of the appropriate sounds. One evening, when all the laboratory personnel had gone home and she was in the lobby of the hospital, the lobby phone rang, and a nurse observed her to have a psychomotor seizure with unconsciousness and groping and grasping movements of her hands.

There can be little doubt that in her own natural environment the sound of telephone bells evoked seizures, but that a startle factor must also be present. When electrodes were in place, she expected the sounds, so the startle factor could not be present, even though the study employed painstaking and time-consuming recording techniques, randomized the presentation of the bells, and even introduced them into music which was being played for her.

E. Major Motor Seizures Evoked by Specific and Nonstartling Sounds

The next patient also had seizures evoked by specific sounds associated with the use of the telephone. All of his seizures were major motor in type. The exact evoking factor could not be detected in the laboratory.

CASE 8. This patient, a thirty-nine-year-old male beauty shop owner, complained of seizures of seven years duration. The first seizure occurred after being struck in the genitalia by a softball. While telephoning his physician for help, he fell to the floor exhibiting tonic and clonic movements. He was weak and tired upon regaining consciousness, without specific symptoms or evidence of incontinence. He was hospitalized, and an electrocardiogram and routine laboratory work were within normal limits. A major motor seizure occurred one week later; the patient fell, lacerating his scalp. Again, there were no localizing symptoms but fatigue and postictal motor aphasia were noted. Carotid arteriogram and pneumoencephalogram were normal. The patient was started on anticonvulsant medication.

Six months later, the patient began to experience major motor seizures ushered in by an aura consisting of a buzzing sound in his ears, lightheadedness, a burnt taste in his mouth, and a generalized feeling that ambient sounds were distant, as if heard from the bottom of a rain barrel. The attacks occurred when answering the telephone. When the phone rang, he would pick it up, begin to talk, and have a seizure. In his attacks the patient was always unconscious, with tonic and clonic movements, and with occasional incontinence and tongue biting. The attacks lasted sixty to ninety seconds and were followed by postictal fatigue and confusion.

The past medical history was noncontributory as were social

and family histories, except that one nephew was mentally retarded and had major motor seizures.

The physical and neurological examinations were normal.

Laboratory studies, including skull X rays and brain scan, were normal. Routine EEGs showed evidence of a nonspecific abnormality in the bisylvian regions, of indeterminate clinical significance. A sleep recording showed no activation of epileptogenic activity or other abnormality. Neuropsychological testing revealed the patient to be functioning in the bright-normal range of intelligence. Other laboratory findings were entirely within normal limits.

After establishment of the baseline values, the patient underwent extensive EEG studies. The tapes used for startle epilepsy did not precipitate seizures or evoke dysrhythmia. He was recorded during all conceivable situations in which a telephone call might evoke one of his seizures. These situations included conversations with multiple individuals both known and unknown to the patient.

It was not possible to evoke a seizure or dysrhythmia in the laboratory. Care was taken to employ for incoming calls the actual telephone instruments used and the voices heard when his seizures had occurred The ultimate in this attempt was accomplished in his place of business. By means of a biopack attached to his chest, his EEG was telemetered to a portable EEG machine in the rear of his shop. He went about his usual chores and received calls on the instrument in the shop and from customers who had initiated calls which had on other occasions resulted in seizures. The same telephone instruments were employed, but seizures were not evoked.

Telephone transmission defects were considered as a possible evoking factor. Presentation of an audio tape compiling these various types of defects, including the rain barrel effect, evoked no clinical or EEG abnormality. This patient had experienced fifteen major seizures, and occasionally, aborted seizures, all related to use of the telephone. He had experienced only one seizure when not telephoning. Despite the failures in the laboratory, this patient should be considered as an instance of auditory-evoked seizures and one in which the stimulus is obscure, but specifically related somehow to telephone transmission.

In 1966, Doctor Jordon Popper of Honolulu informed the author of a serviceman seen at Trippler Army Hospital who had seizures evoked by the sounds of billiard balls clicking. On neurological evaluation he was found to have signs of a temporal lobe brain tumor, and, on exploration, an astrocytoma was found and removed. His seizures did not recur, thus he was not available for study. While this patient was not studied in detail as an example of reflex epilepsy (the presence of the brain tumor placed such observations in a secondary role), he may well be another example of the role of specific sounds.

F. Seizures Evoked by Nonspecific and Startling Voices

More complex is the next patient whose seizures were evoked by certain sounds—voices, apparently those of someone in command. A startling effect was necessary, and the patient had to be concentrating on some task.

CASE 9.   This thirty-seven-year-old, married, female hydraulic engineer had her first seizure at twelve years of age. Her seizures occurred when she was concentrating on mental problems and was startled by someone, usually a male, briskly calling her name. She could often abort the seizure by concentration. In this way, at work she could delay the phenomenon long enough to walk to the ladies room. She would then often have a major motor seizure lasting about five minutes, many times with urinary incontinence. The seizures were followed by a twenty-minute period of euphoria and confusion. She had many seizures in high school and college, and estimated that she has had approximately fifty major motor seizures in her lifetime. She had five major motor seizures and eight to nine dream states or aborted seizures in the year prior to study.

The patient's father (sixty-four years old) had two or three seizures when he was thirty-five years old, but has had none since being maintained on low doses of phenobarbital. The patient's sister (now thirty-eight years old) had two seizures at twelve years of age and one at thirty-six years of age. The patient's son (now fourteen years old) has had two seizures.

The patient reported in relating her medical history that at one year of age, she had a high fever of unknown origin (her sister and father were similarly ill at the same time).

The physical examination was negative except for mild *pectus escavatum* deformity. The neurological examination was also normal, as were routine laboratory and X-ray studies.

All of her EEGs were normal except one record which was taken postictally and which suggested potential epileptogenic activity symmetrical in both hemispheres. Neuropsychological testing was unremarkable.

In this patient, seizures could not be evoked in the Research Laboratory. Her employer recorded on tape for us the brusque command, "Bev, I want you to do this right away," and similar commands. While she was concentrating in the EEG laboratory on the intricacies of operating a new computation machine with which she was unfamiliar, this tape recording was introduced over the speaker system but without effect. While she was engaged in typing a manuscript, various staff members abruptly broke into the laboratory giving the same brusque commands, again without effect.

It was thought up to this point that only male voices evoked her seizures. However, the only seizure evoked during hospitalization was during the neuropsychological testing and, unfortunately, this was without EEG recording. The seizure occurred when the neuropsychology technician (female) gave a rather brusque command while the patient was concentrating deeply upon a test. The technician said, "Bev, let's turn to this now," and a definite major motor seizure occurred with the postictal EEG changes noted above. On the following day, the situation was recreated in the Epilepsy Research Laboratory with the same technician, with the same neuropsychology equipment. At the same point in the neuropsychological testing, the same brusque command was given but no seizure or dysrhythmia was evoked.

In this patient a startling effect was necessary; a human voice, either male or female, uttering a command, comprised the evoking stimulus. The stimulus was not effective unless the patient was in deep concentration.

G.   *Aphasic and Major Motor Seizures Evoked by Nonstartling and Specific Voices*

CASE 10. This patient has been previously reported by Forster et al.[15] She was a fifty-three-year-old married woman who had been involved in an automobile accident in 1944 and had suffered a severe head injury. She was unconscious for four days and approximately two years later developed seizures. These were of two different types. The first type consisted of major motor convulsions without a well-defined aura, ushered in with a cry, followed by unconsciousness and tonic-clonic movements. Tongue biting and postictal confusion were occasionally noted.

The second type of attack was described as a "funny feeling," a momentary sensation of inactivity in which she dropped objects from her hand and had some mouthing movements, followed by a period of several minutes in which she could not speak. These focal seizures occurred almost exclusively while listening to the radio. She was aware that the voices of three particular radio announcers evoked the seizures. Occasionally, voices in stores and other public places also evoked the attacks, but these voices were difficult to identify.

She had been placed on sodium diphenylhydantoin, 300 mg per day, in about 1947 and had taken this regularly until 1961. At that time, dosage was increased to 400 mg per day and primidone, 500 mg per day, was added. The major motor seizures continued at an approximate frequency of three to four per month, and the temporal lobe seizures occurred at a rate of from four per week to three per day. During this interim, she had been treated with mephenytoin (Mesantoin®) and Riker 594 without effect. Nitrazepam (Mogadon®, LA-1), 15 mg per day, was added on November 23, 1965, and no major seizures occurred subsequently, although the focal seizures persisted at the above-reported frequency.

During previous hospitalizations for attempts at seizure control, the following additional diagnoses had been made: diabetes mellitus (adult onset), pernicious anemia, cholelithiasis, vitiligo, and primidone-induced dermatitis medicamentosa.

The family history revealed a sister with diabetes, and the mother and one brother with vitiligo. There was no family history of seizures.

On physical examination, generalized vitiligo was noted and there were burn scars at the right breast and right wrist, with donor skin graft sites at the right thigh. Burns had occurred during major motor seizures.

Neurological examination was negative except for decreased ankle jerks bilaterally and symmetrically.

Routine laboratory studies were normal except that the chest X rays revealed mild pulmonary emphysema.

Numerous routine electroencephalograms in sleep, waking, isolation, and with photic and pattern stimulation over a fifteen-year period were normal. Pneumoencephalography in 1951 and 1962 indicated cortical atrophy, greater on the left side.

In this patient, detailed studies were undertaken to determine whether or not her seizures were voice-induced. These studies are described in some detail since she is the only patient in the literature with this problem.

RESEARCH STUDIES

The three radio announcers supplied us with tapes of their radio programs. These programs were of newscasts and of the usual type of Midwestern exchange or sales programs, listing names of objects for sale and exchange, along with telephone numbers. When the patient listened to these tapes in the laboratory, seizures and EEG changes were evoked, as shown in Table V. A reasonable spacing of time between the days of presentations of the suspected stimuli was arranged to avoid a conditioning effect during the period of study. With the presentation of announcers on the local radio station in Madison, and upon hearing the voices of the scientists in the laboratory of the Epilepsy Center, no seizure and no dysrhythmia occurred. The three announcers to whom the patient knew she was sensitive are listed as R.Z., E.D. and R.H. They broadcast over radio stations in Waupun, Fond du Lac, and Milwaukee, Wisconsin. The studies were begun with the tape of announcer R.Z.'s program, and the patient was conditioned (see Chapter 12) to the tape before being exposed to the other two tapes. This probably explains why responses to the other two announcers were less severe.

Seizures occurred eighteen times in the laboratory (Fig. 16)

TABLE V

STUDY OF VOICE-EVOKED EPILEPSY

Date	Patient's State	Stimulus Presented	Clinical Response	EEG Response
11- 1-67	Awake-resting	Local radio announcers	O	N
11- 1-67	Awake-resting	R.Z. tape 1	Focal seizure	Left temporal dysrhythmia
11- 1-67	Awake-resting	Audiovisual tape of R.Z. tape 1	O	N
11- 1-67	Awake-resting	Continuation of R.Z. tape 1	Focal seizure	Left temporal dysrhythmia
11- 8-67	Awake-resting	Local radio announcers	O	N
11- 8-67	Awake-resting	R.Z. tape 1	Focal seizure	Left temporal dysrhythmia
11- 8-67	Awake-resting	Repeat above	O	N
11- 8-67	Awake-resting	Continuation of R.Z. tape 1	Focal seizure (slight)	Left temporal dysrhythmia
11-14-67	Awake-resting	Local radio	O	N
11-14-67	Awake-resting	R.Z. tape 1	Focal seizure	Left temporal dysrhythmia
11-14-67	Awake-resting	Replay above, X2	O	N
11-15-67	Awake-resting	E.D. tape	O	N
11-16-67	Hypnosis	Told to have seizure (R.Z. suggested)	Focal seizure	N
11-20-67	Simulated seizure	None	Seizure	N
--	Hyperventilation	None	O	N
--	Induced sleep	R.Z. tape 1	Focal seizure	Left temporal dysrhythmia
11-24-67	Awake-resting, with anticonvulsants reduced	Local radio announcers	O	N
--	Awake-resting, with anticonvulsants reduced	R.Z. tape 1	Focal to grand mal seizure	Left temporal dysrhythmia (generalized)
--	Awake-resting, with anticonvulsants reduced	Continuation of R.Z. tape 1	Focal to grand mal seizure	Left temporal dysrhythmia (generalized)
11-29-67	Awake-resting, conditioned to R.Z. tape 1	E.D. tape	Focal seizure (slight)	Left temporal dysrhythmia
--	Conditioned to E.D. tape	R.H. tape	Aura	O dysrhythmia

From Forster, F. M., Hansotia, P., Cleeland, C. S., and Ludwig, A.: A case of voice-induced epilepsy treated by conditioning. *Neurology, 19:*325, 1969.

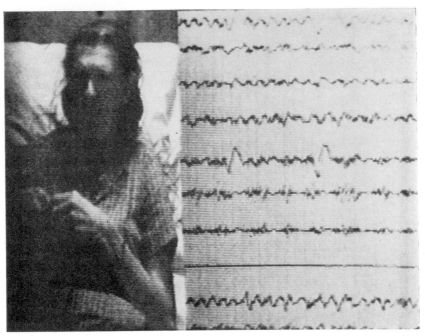

Figure 16.   From AV tape. Patient in aphasic seizure, attempting to communicate by gesturing. EEG shows spiking dysrhythmia, most prominent in left anterior temporal lead (second channel from bottom). Reprinted from *Physiological Effects of Noise*, Plenum Press, 1970.

but only upon presentation of the radio announcers' taped voices. In the seizures, the patient would frown and place either hand (usually her right) to her jaw, with her head slanting to the left. There was some quivering of the jaw and no response occurred to such questions as "Are you all right?" The patient was given verbal or numerical signs which she could not later recall, thus indicating an interruption of consciousness, and she would begin to vocalize "Ah, ah, ah, ah," as in a form of arrested speech. This lasted from thirty seconds to one minute, and the patient was quite distraught.

Following this, she had amnestic aphasia lasting from three to five minutes. She could, on command, identify the nature of objects and indicate their function, but she could not recall their names. When given the name of an object in a series of nouns, she could identify the correct name. When shown a penknife, she made a whittling movement with her fingers; when shown scissors, she made a scissoring movement with her fingers. She was unable to state a name, but identified the given object when it was presented in a list of other nouns. The aphasia was present in both of her languages, English and German. On command, she could choose one object from many, and she could write very laboriously. She could comprehend and carry out written commands such as "close your eyes."

The seizures could be evoked by the noxious voices with the patient in either a waking-resting state or in drug-induced sleep. Hyperventilation did not evoke the seizures. During hypnosis, a seizure was induced when the patient was told that she was listening to R.Z. and told to have a seizure. This was a true seizure, virtually identical with her usual and customary attacks and followed by the post-seizure aphasia which persisted into the post hypnotic state, despite the suggestion that she would be normal upon completion of hypnosis. The seizure, however, was not accompanied by an evident EEG dysrhythmia. Several days later the patient was requested to simulate a seizure, but she could not do this accurately. She could not imitate the aphasic component nor was she aware of the brief loss of consciousness in her seizure.

The patient's anticonvulsant medications were withheld for twenty-four hours in order to make the EEG dysrhythmia more evident, particularly in the hope of finding the primary electrical discharge. Presentation of the noxious voice on two occasions then induced focal seizures which proceeded into major motor seizures.

The evaluation of the voice-induced EEG dysrhythmia was an integral part of the study of this patient. The patient's resting record and sleep records were normal, as was the record obtained in sensory restriction. EEGs during presentation of other voices were also normal. EEG dysrhythmias occurred therefore only in association with the presentation of the particular voices. The dysrthymia began in the left temporal lobe, as indicated by the tracings from the ear electrode and from electrodes placed in the midtemporal region. The dysrhythmia during the focal seizures registered as slow 4- to 6-cycles-per-second sharp waves, developing into sharp spiking discharges. These, however, were apparent only after the patient had experienced a warning and was in the process of having a seizure. New arrangements of electrodes failed to display the primary spiking discharge. When the patient's anticonvulsant medications were reduced and the focal seizures proceeded into major convulsions, the theta activity became sharper and evolved into sharp spiking discharges with a generalized spread; but again, the primary dysrhythmia was not apparent.

An audio tape was made by each of the three announcers, and a single paragraph was chosen for voice analysis. This was read by each of the announcers in multiple presentations so that there was a total of six presentations by the three specific radio announcers whose voices induced seizures. Additional recordings were made of ten voices which had failed to evoke any dysrhythmia. These included male scientists who had worked with the patient in the Epilepsy Center Laboratories and other radio announcers. The recordings were sent to a voice print laboratory for a printout of the frequencies. Analysis of these prints did not establish any specific characteristic frequency which was limited to the six recordings by the three announcers. When the prints were divided into groups, using the double blind technique, no absolute clear distinction between the characteristics of the noxious and the innocuous voices was found either by Doctor Kersta of the voice print laboratory or by any of the physicians conducting the study; however, the analysis suggests that the noxious factors might lay in a low index of average pitch frequency and the time rate of change in speech formats and syllabic rates.

The study of the voice prints suggests that an element of prosody may play a role. Monrad-Krohn[19] defines prosody as a variation of pitch, rhythm, and stress of pronunciation.

The elusiveness of the nature of the evoking stimulus in certain kinds of reflex epilepsy is well illustrated in this case. Review of the AV tapes disclosed no common word, phrase, number or sound as clearly representing the evoking stimulus in the announcers' recordings. In reviewing the AV tapes, it was obvious that the patient's seizures did not occur at the same places in the audio tapes. Moreover, when the same text was read by one of the laboratory staff members no seizures occurred. The evoking factor existed in the voices of the announcers and was more subtle than the words themselves.

The ten patients described in this chapter demonstrate the wide variations in auditory-induced epilepsy. The variations included those of the stimuli and of the responses. The stimuli varied widely in their specificity or lack of specificity and in the role of surprise or startle. The responses to the stimuli also varied greatly. The seizure types ranged from myoclonus to major motor seizures.

There was considerable variation in the intellectual accomplishments of the patients, with the most severe intellectual involvement present in those patients activated by the least specific stimulus. A major motor seizure evoked by any loud, sudden noise occurred in the patient with the greatest intellectual deficit. A very specific stimulus (a voice with authority), under the most rigorous situations of deep concentration evoked seizures in the patient with the greatest intellectual achievements. The patient with the most specific stimulus (certain voices), and evoked aphasic seizures, had suffered some intellectual impairment as a result of the head injury which gave rise to her seizures.

Musicogenic epilepsy is of a far different nature than the aforementioned types of epilepsy. This opinion is shared by Gastaut and Privano,[9] and Peet, Daly, and Bickford.[12] Pescher and Rollin[18] point out that the reflex is more complex in musicogenic epilepsy, and that it is not completely understood. They feel that the rare occurrence of pure audiogenic seizures in man is due to the small ecologic importance of the cortical representation of tone in comparison to the higher associative areas of auditory function in the human. For these reasons, musicogenic epilepsy is dealt with in the next chapter.

REFERENCES

1. Gowers, W. G.: *Epilepsy and Other Chronic Convulsive Diseases.* J. London and A. Churchill, 1901, p. 108.
2. Thomas, A.: A propos de l'epilepsie reflexes. *Presse Med,* 47:1467, 1939.

3. Critchley, M.: Uber Reflex-Epilepsie, *Schweiz Arch Neurol Neurochir Psychiat*, 35:256, 1935.
4. Strauss, H.: Jacksonian seizures of reflex origin. *Arch Neurol Psychiat*, 44:140, 1940.
5. Allen, J. M.: Observations on cases of reflex epilepsy. *N Z Med J*, 44:135, 1945.
6. Kliemann, F. D. and Ferreira, N. P.: Sobressalto patologico; aspectos clinicos e electroencefalograficos. *Arch Neuro-Psiquait* (S. Paulo), 25:130, 1967.
7. Cohen, N. M., McAuliffe, M., and Aird, R. B.: Startle epilepsy treated with chlordiaze poxice. *Dis Nerv Syst*, 22:20, 1961.
8. Strobos, R. J.: Acousticomotor seizures. *Electroencephalogr Clin Neurophysiol*, 14:129, 1962.
9. Gastaut, H. and Privano, E.: Epilepsia indotta da simulazione undivita intermittente rimica O epilessia psofogenica. *Arch N Picol Neurol Psychiat*, 10:297, 1949.
10. Gastaut, H., Roger, J., Corrici, J., and Gastaut, Y.: Epilepsy induced by rhythmic intermittent auditory stimulation or epilepsy "posphogenique." *Electroencephalogr Clin Neurophysiol*, 1:121, 1949.
11. Booker, H., Forster, F., and Klove, H.: Extinction factors in acousticomotor seizures. *Neurology*, 15:1095, 1965.
12. Peet, R. M., Daly, D., and Bickford, R. G.: Some clinical and electroencephalographic responses to sound stimulation in epileptic patients. *Trans Am Neurol Assoc*, 77:215, 1952.
13. Foerster, O.: Die Pathogenesis des epilepileptischen Anfalls. *Dtsch Ztschr Nervenhlk*, 94:15, 1926.
14. Forster, F. M.: Epilepsia del lóbulo temporal. *Arch Médicos de Cuba*, 3:252, 1952.
15. Forster, F. M., Hansotia, P., Cleeland, C. S., and Ludwig, A.: A case of voice-induced epilepsy treated by conditioning. *Neurology*, 19:325, 1969.
16. Wabayashi, J., Kurita, H., and Yoshida, J.: A case of startle epilepsy. *Psychiat Neurol Japan*, 64:1101, 1962.
17. Taylor, S.: A case of musicogenic epilepsy. *J R Nav Med Serv*, 28:394, 1942.
18. Pascher, W. and Rollin, H.: Akustiche Reflexepilepsien. *Nervenarzt*, 41:68, 1970.
19. Monrad-Krohn, G. J.: *The third element of speech: prosody and its disorders in problems of dynamic neurology*. L. Halpern (Ed.), Jerusalem, 1963. New York, Grune and Stratton.
20. Forster, F. M.: Human studies of epileptic seizures induced by sound and their conditioned extinction. In Welch, B. L. and Welch, A. S. (Eds.): *Physiological Effects of Noise*, New York, London, Plenum Pr, 1970, p. 151.

CHAPTER 4

MUSICOGENIC EPILEPSY

Musicogenic epilepsy could be considered a form of auditory-evoked epilepsy. However, the theme of the music usually produces the seizures rather than the specific sounds, and there may even be an important factor in the memory components while listening to the music. These facts suggest that musicogenic epilepsy might well be a communication disorder, albeit nonverbal, and therefore a disorder of a higher cognitive function.[1] Therefore, it is appropriate to treat this entity separately since the seizure evocation is highly complex.

The first case of musicogenic epilepsy was described in 1884 by Merzheevski.[2] After this, cases appeared sporadically in the literature until 1937 when Critchley published the first series of cases and delineated the condition.[3] There are now approximately fifty cases in the world literature. Titeca,[4] Weber,[5] Joynt, Green, and Green,[6] Poskanzer, Brown, and Miller,[7] and Pascher and Rollin[8] have written careful reviews of literature.

CASES OF MUSICOGENIC EPILEPSY

Nine patients with a possible diagnosis of musicogenic epilepsy were referred to the University of Wisconsin laboratory for study. In five of these patients the diagnosis was confirmed.

The case summaries of the five patients with musicogenic epilepsy follow:

CASE 1. This patient, a thirty-six-year-old, married, unemployed male had seizures beginning at age seventeen while working as an usher in a movie theater. At first he experienced a generalized numbness and tingling throughout his body and a *deja vu* phenomenon. He was vaguely aware that when listening to his own musical records he occasionally had these episodes of tingling and *deja vu* phenomenon and thought the episodes might have lasted a minute or so. At age twenty-three, the seizures began to last longer and were more complex in their content. Following the generalized numbness, tingling, and *deja vu* phenomenon, the patient would stare, make smacking movements with his lips, moisten his lips with his tongue, flex his arms across his chest, sometimes make growling noises, slowly slide to the floor if he was standing, or if seated, he would slump forward in his chair. This would be followed by prolonged periods of automatisms and inability to name objects. This gradually developing change in seizure pattern made the attacks more apparent to others. During this period his wife became aware of the fact that music precipitated his seizures. The incidence of these seizures varied from one per day over three consecutive days to one every two weeks.

In addition to the psychomotor seizures, the patient had major motor seizures with head deviation to the left which also began at age twenty-three.

These were at first nocturnal. He began having occasional diurnal major motor seizures, but these were invariably preceded by the generalized numbness, tingling and *deja vu* phenomenon, and may have been precipitated by music.

Anticonvulsant medication controlled the major motor seizures but did not effect the incidence of the temporal lobe musico-genic seizures.

Review of systems and family history were negative. Physical and neurological examinations were normal. Laboratory studies, including pneumoencephalogram and angiogram, were normal, except for a slight asymmetry in the internal cerebral vein on the left which was not felt to be significant. The remainder of the laboratory examinations were normal. Resting and sleep electroencephalographic studies were normal except for some slight but consistent slowing in the left temporal area, with occasional theta activity.

On one occasion, while in the hospital and when performing his morning ablutions, the patient was unaware that a radio was being played softly in an adjoining room. Despite his unawareness, a typical psychomotor seizure was evoked by the appropriate music.

CASE 2. This patient, a thirty-six-year-old wife of a sergeant, was referred from an Army base in Texas because of the onset of seizures at age thirty-five. The original seizure was nocturnal, major motor in type. This was followed by almost daily brief episodes lasting only a few seconds and consisting of the feeling that she "was someone else." She has had only one subsequent major motor seizure when her medication was interrupted for a pelvic surgical procedure. Later in these minor seizures, she had in addition a strange taste in her mouth and was noted to stare transiently. Her husband noted that these occurred only while she was listening to western music played over the local radio station, or to tapes he had made of these broadcasts.

Family and past history were noncontributory. Physical and neurological examinations were negative, except for a slight reflex asymmetry with the deep tendon reflexes being greater on the left. There was impaired sound localization in the left auditory fields. Laboratory studies were normal, including brain scan and pneumoencephalogram. EEGs in the resting, sleep, and sensory-deprived state were normal.

CASE 3. This patient, a forty-eight-year old female, frequently "passed out" while playing the church organ at age ten and consequently had to stop this endeavor. About age twenty-seven, she began experiencing one to two times weekly, episodes consisting of an aura in which warmth would spread from her toes to her chest, followed by loss of consciousness of thirty to sixty seconds duration, then by a desire to sleep for a few minutes. Her sister observed several of these episodes and described them as follows: "she would clasp her hands as if in prayer and slump in her chair or sometimes fall down." Medication did not control these episodes. Approximately twelve years prior to admission, in 1954, the patient's sister discovered a relationship between the seizures and music. When the patient attended on four different occasions a particular church service, each time suffering a seizure, her sister became aware of the role of music in precipitating the seizures.

The patient's seizures were characterized by a loss of awareness of her surroundings without a preceding aura except for the thought "isn't this music nice." Her sister observed smacking of the lips during these episodes which lasted up to a minute. The episodes were followed by confusion and asking "what has happened and where am I?" At no time was there any incontinence, muscle stiffness, jerking movements, or tongue biting. The patient and her sister were unable to relate her seizures to any specific type of music or any specific instrumentation. Since noting the relationship between music and seizures and accordingly avoiding music, the number of seizures had decreased to one to two per month and were almost always precipitated by inadvertently heard music. Her social life was severely curtailed in that she went nowhere where music might be heard. Adequate dosages of appropriate anticonvulsants failed to control the seizures.

Past history and family history were noncontributory except that a brother, age forty-five, had febrile convulsions as a child as well as seizures following an accident at age three. This history was complicated by the fact that he apparently had a tumor removed at age six and required further surgery at age twenty-four for "brain scars." He has been seizure free since age twenty-seven. Physical and neurological examinations were normal except for thyrotoxic exophthalmos. Laboratory studies included audiometric testing which revealed normal hearing levels. X rays of the skull were negative. Neuropsychological testing indicated mild impairment of adaptive abilities. The usual laboratory examinations, including routine EEGs, were within normal limits.

CASE 4. This patient, a thirty-seven-year-old white male, had experienced seizures for twenty years. His first seizure was major motor in type. Since this initial episode, seizures have been recurrent and either major motor or psychomotor in type. The patient's wife made the observation eight years ago that seizure activity appeared to be triggered by music. The most common seizure type occurred once or twice per month; it was characterized by a brief aura of nonspecific anxiety and a feeling of "a shade coming down over my eyes." Following this, automatic behavior such as walking or repeating fragments of previously performed purposeful behavior frequently occurred. Abnormal lip and tongue movements were noted during these periods. The episodes were usually followed by pounding bilateral headache, with increased sensitivity to light but not to sound. The patient had been evaluated by a number of physicians and since age twenty had been taking appropriate anticonvulsants in increasing dosages. He had no further major motor seizures, but these medications did not control the minor seizures. At age thirty-two, brain scan, skull X rays, left carotid angiogram, and pneumoencephalogram were reported to have been within normal limits. His most recent seizure was induced by music while passing through O'Hare Airport in Chicago on the way to Madison, Wisconsin from his home in New Jersey.

The patient was trained and had been employed as a high school teacher. But two years ago, he was asked to leave his job because of seizures, and had not worked since. He described decrease in pleasurable activities and episodes of frank depression, without suicidal ideation, over the past five or six years. He had had a course of psychotherapy without change in his mental outlook or seizure frequency.

Past medical history revealed no history of significant trauma (including birth), serious illnesses or operations, allergies, or transfusions. Irregular areas of vitiliginous depigmentation of the skin have been present since birth. The father and grandfather have a similar syndrome. Family history was negative for neurological disease. Physical and neurological examinations were normal. Admission blood and urine laboratory studies were normal except for eosinophilia. The patient's skull and chest X rays were normal. Routine EEGs were normal.

CASE 5. This patient was a thirty-five-year-old housewife who at age twenty-two, after a spontaneous abortion, had a generalized tonic-clonic seizure followed by a similar episode four months later. EEG, pneumoencephalogram, and carotid angiography were reported as normal. She was begun on anticonvulsant medication but continued to have seizures. Major motor seizures were no longer present, but minor seizures characterized by staring episodes with altered consciousness and without any tonic-clonic activity persisted, occurring about once a month. The seizures lasted approximately three to five minutes, were occasionally associated with urinary incontinence, and were followed by a period of postictal confusion. Her husband became aware of the fact that these seizures occurred while listening to music.

General physical and neurological examinations were normal except for hypertension, and this was found to be due to renal artery occlusive disease. Routine EEGs were normal.

Table VI summarizes some of the clinical aspects of these five patients. There is no significant sex difference in this series, nor has any been noted in the literature. Although all of the patients were in middle life when studied, four of the patients' seizures had been present for long periods of time (seventeen to thirty years).

The early age of onset (ten years) in Case 3 is significant in that she is the only one of the patients studied who had been a musician and at that age was seriously studying the piano. She therefore had created significant musical engrams.

Of greater significance is the long duration of the illness before the diagnosis was made. Case 2 is an exception in this regard, for she had experienced seizures for only six months before the diagnosis of musicogenic epilepsy was made. This was due to the fact that her husband played tapes of the noxious music, and undoubtedly, the association of seizure occurrence with his motor activity in handling the tape recorder led to the early diagnosis. The long delay in diagnosis in the other four patients (four to twenty-six years) was due at least in part to the amount of music exposure to which these patients were subjected. All of them liked music and played records, tapes, or the radio almost incessantly before the diagnosis was made. Music became an almost constant part of their daily milieu; therefore the occurrence of seizures was not immediately linked to the stimulus. Moreover, it was in all five cases the relatives, not the patients, who made the diagnosis. This is in part due to the postictal confusion. When the seizure and postictal state were completed, the study patients were unable to recall what music had been playing immediately prior to the seizure evocation, thus suggesting a retrograde amnesia.

The occurrence of musicogenic epilepsy is unrelated to the patient's musical ability. The patients may be accomplished

TABLE VI

CLINICAL AND LABORATORY DATA—CASES OF MUSICOGENIC EPILEPSY

Case Number	Age	Age of Onset	Duration Before Noted	Sex	Family History	Music Sophisti- cation	Hand	Dominance Eye	Foot	Routine EEG
1	34	17	4 yrs.	M	0	0	R	L	R	Mild theta—L.T.
2	36	36	6 mos.	F	0	0	L	L	R	N
3	48	10	26 yrs.	F	+	++++	R	R	R	N
4	37	17	9 yrs.	M	0	++	R	R	R	N
5	35	22	12 yrs.	F	0	0	R	L	R	N

musicians, as in the case of Strang[13] and in Case 3. The ability varies to the opposite extreme, as shown in Case 1, who not only had difficulty in recognizing the sound of particular instruments but sometimes could not reliably distinguish organ music from orchestral renditions. Musicians with musicogenic epilepsy may evoke their seizures by playing an instrument[12] (and also Case 3). Piotrokowsky[14] reported a patient with musicogenic epilepsy who evoked his seizures by singing while intoxicated. This component of singing introduces the factor of language or communication epilepsy in its broader connotation.

While alcohol can be a precipitant of seizures in some patients, it is not a significant or frequent factor in musicogenic epilepsy. In another case that the author had studied, which was reported by Lennox,[15] the patient felt that a few drinks made him more susceptible to the deleterious effects of music. This patient, who was a physician and also a musician, accidentally self-induced a psychomotor seizure while playing the organ for the annual Christmas caroling in his home town. While in the midst of a solemn hymn, he had a psychomotor seizure during which he rendered "hot jazz" for several minutes. He had a total amnesia on regaining consciousness, but the effect on the community was startling! In the late 1940s, the author studied him extensively in the EEG laboratory at the Jefferson Hospital, Philadelphia but was unable to induce a seizure in the laboratory setting. He was presented with a wide selection of music, including anything he thought might evoke a seizure. Since his seizures often occurred when he was relaxed, had had a few drinks of bourbon, and was listening to his records, this situation was recreated in the laboratory, but no seizures could be elicited.

Heredity plays little or no role in musicogenic epilepsy. The family histories of four of the study's patients were entirely negative for seizure disorders. In the third case, a brother had had a febrile convulsion and later had posttraumatic epilepsy. There were no other seizure manifestations in her direct or collateral lines. Reifenberg[16] studied twins. One of them had musicogenic epilepsy, but the other had no seizures. The role of heredity in musicogenic epilepsy must be negligible if present at all.

The five patients with musicogenic epilepsy had normal EEGs in the resting, sleep, and sensory-deprived states. Case 1 had some mild theta activity in his left temporal leads when not exposed to music, but this was not epileptogenic.

RESEARCH STUDIES

Musicogenic epilepsy is more complex than many of the other forms of reflex epilepsy. It is therefore not possible to devise a standard testing battery which will serve the entire group as satisfactorily as in some forms of reflex epilepsy, e.g. the visually induced epilepsies. The problems in musicogenic epilepsy require more individualization. However, some semblance of a standard approach is possible, at least for the original survey for music which will induce seizures in the individual patient. The survey also serves the purpose of eliminating from consideration types of music which do not evoke seizures. Types of music which do not evoke seizures can be listened to by the patient without fear of seizures. This determination is of value to the patients, for they have been musically deprived and have avoided music, including that which is perfectly safe for them.

The audio tapes used for screening, or surveying, were designed so as to include a broad range of music. For example, the first one presented to the patients with possible musicogenic epilepsy begins with Tchaikovsky's *1812 Overture,* moves through college band numbers which approach jazz, into New Orleans Jazz, and then into Rock and Roll music. Other screening tapes allow further exploration into popular music of the mid-nineteen thirties, into the semiclassical music such as the Strauss Waltzes, into a broad selection of ballets, overtures and symphonies at one end of the spectrum, and at the other end, transitional and "hard" Rock and Roll. Attention was also given to Oriental and primitive music as well as seasonal music (for example, Christmas carols). The recorded music also ranged from single instrument and computer-simulated music to full orchestrations, both with and without vocal renditions.

Each of the five patients, when presented in the laboratory with the scanning tapes and further explorations as noted above, had on repeated occasions seizures and definite epileptogenic abnormalities. Table VII presents pertinent clinical and research findings on these patients.

The seizures observed in the laboratory upon presentation of music were all psychomotor (partial complex) and quite stereotyped for each patient and indeed were quite similar in all patients (Fig. 17). The patients showed lip smacking and mouthing movements. Early in the onset of the seizures, the patients would turn their heads from side to side, fumble with their clothes, and produce objects, such as cigarettes or note paper and pencil, from their pockets. They did not respond to questions or verbal commands in the early part of the seizure. They later would respond with questions as "what?" or statements as "I can't understand you," suggesting an aphasic component. They attempted to remove the electrodes and, on occasion, when restrained from leaving the EEG chair, would strike out or kick at the physician or technician. The seizures lasted from three to ten minutes. Postictally the patients were confused and had no recollection of the events of the seizure.

The first patient had twenty-seven seizures in the laboratory which were essentially identical. The large number of seizures induced in this patient was due to two facts; (a) the attempt of the study to determine all the musical numbers which evoked seizures in him in the search for a commonality of stimuli, and (b) the lack of understanding as to how best to treat this kind of epilepsy. Each of the other four patients had no more than five seizures.

The evoking factor in the music stimulus in our patients was not related to the mechanics of music but rather to the theme. It was impossible to determine any particular note, chord, or instrumentation that evoked the epileptogenic activity.

The audiovisual tapes of the first musicogenic patient were reviewed by members of the faculty of the School of Music of the University of Wisconsin. At the moment of occurrence of the anterior temporal lobe spiking dysrhythmia, the instruments, notes, chords, and key were identified, but no common musical denominator was identified. Moreover in these patients, the audiovisual tape recordings were played for the patient and,

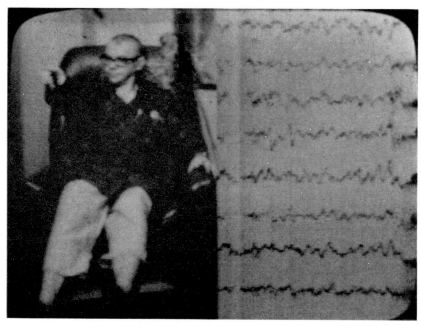

Figure 17. Musicogenic epilepsy. Case 4. Seizure evoked by Rock and Roll music. Patient is gesticulating and crying out, purposefully but irrelevantly. EEG shows spiking dysrhythmia from left anterior temporal leads (fourth and sixth channels of EEG from top).

while listening to the music from the speaker, a second EEG was obtained. There was no correlation in the time of appearance of the dysrhythmia in the two EEGs. Therefore, a mechanical musical factor is most unlikely.

The specificity of the evoking stimulus lies in the theme or type of music rather than in the mechanics of the presentation. In each patient, a specificity for the type of music which evoked these seizures was noted. Professors McPeek and Moser of the Music Department of the University of Wisconsin, upon reviewing the data on the first patient, concluded that the type of music which affected the patient "was music derived from the post-romantic tradition of Western art music, specifically embodying the shifting complex of lush harmonies as evidenced in the music of Debussy and Sibelius."

In the second patient, the only type of music which evoked

seizures was cowboy-western music, and this occurred on the type of presentation which is customarily played live over the radio stations in the southwestern part of the United States. The more sophisticated albums of cowboy-western music did not affect her.

In the third patient, the Strauss waltzes, Tchaikovsky's ballets, parts of Handel's *Messiah,* and certain Christmas carols as well as parts of *The Sound of Music* and similar musical numbers evoked dysrhythmias and seizures.

The fourth patient had seizures to jazz, rock and roll, and some Oriental types of music. The fifth patient had seizures to cowboy-western and popular ballad music, and to certain church hymns.

The third patient, herself a musician, commented that she felt the problem lay not in the instrumentation but rather in the theme of the music. This of course is quite in accord with the observations made in the course of the study.

In addition to the theme of the music, memory patterns may also play a role. In the laboratory, especially in the first patient, during the two or three seconds immediately after completion of a musical number which had evoked temporal lobe spiking, the spiking dysrhythmia continued, although without a clinical seizure.

The occurrence of spiking discharges immediately after the conclusion of a particularly stirring number is at the time when the music is, according to the patient, "ringing in my ears," and there is somewhat of an "after image" of the music of the concluding bars. This suggests that the music reverberating in the memory circuits may still evoke seizures. It may well be that the evoking stimulus is a complex one, consisting of the input of particular theme factors of music being heard at the moment, plus those factors reverberating in memory circuits. The reports of patients who could induce seizures by recalling appropriate music from memory further this concept.[9, 10]

The presentation of the specific evoking music for the particular patient produced a sharp spiking epileptogenic discharge in the left anterior temporal region in the first (Fig. 18), fourth, and fifth patients, and in the right anterior temporal in the

TABLE VII

EFFECT OF MUSIC ON MUSICOGENIC PATIENTS

Case Number	Type of Music	Type of Seizure Evoked	Type EEG Evoked	Location
1	Popular Mid-30's Ex. "Stardust"	Psychomotor	Spiking discharge Single or electrical seizure	Lt. A.T. (rarely Rt. A.T.)
2	Cowboy-western	Psychomotor	Spiking discharge Single or electrical seizure	Rt. A.T.
3	Classic and Semiclassic Ex. Straus Waltzes Handel's Messiah	Psychomotor	Spiking discharge Single or electrical seizure	Rt. A.T. (occ. Lt. A.T.)
4	Jazz, Rock and Roll Primitive music	Psychomotor	Spiking seizure discharge	Lt. A.T. (occ. Rt. A.T.)
5	Western—Modern Popular music Some church music	Psychomotor	Spiking seizure discharge	L.T.

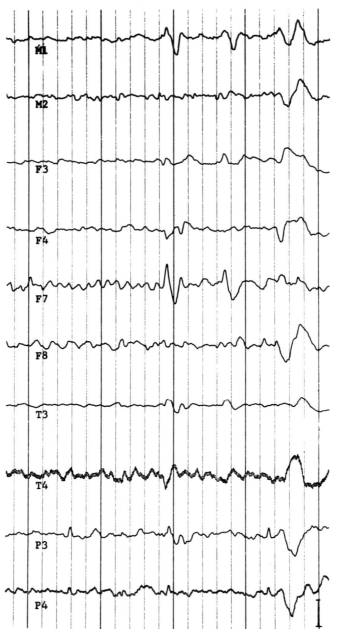

Figure 18. Musicogenic epilepsy. Case 1. Left anterior temporal (F7) spiking dysrhythmia associated with aura. This was the most frequently evoked dysrhythmia in this patient and was often followed by after-discharge and spread of dysrhythmia with clinical seizure.

second and third patients. The first, third, and fourth patients, on rare occasions while listening to the appropriate music, also showed spiking discharges independently and from the opposite temporal lobes (Fig. 19). At no time did these contralateral dysrhythmias proceed into a generalized dysrhythmia, nor were they accompanied by clinical seizures.

When the temporal lobe single spiking dysrhythmia proceeded into a clinical seizure, there could be intervals of six to thirty seconds during which the EEG was normal. A gradual buildup of sharp waves occurred at the same focus as the original spike, followed by spread to other cortical areas and the appearance of the typical seizure (Fig. 20). Shaw and Hill[11] have also commented upon this delay. This delay and subsequent discharge occurred even if the stimulum presentation was halted at the appearance of the temporal lobe spiking discharge.

It should be noted that some correlation existed between cerebral dominance and the laterality of the EEG focus. In Case 3, the left hemisphere appeared dominant, and the EEG focus was right temporal lobe in origin. Handedness, however, in the other four patients correlated quite well with the spiking discharges occurring in the dominant hemisphere (Tables VI and VII). From the data gathered in the study, no final conclusion can be drawn regarding the role of the dominant hemisphere in musicogenic epilepsy, but the evidence is suggestive that musicogenic epilepsy may be a process of the dominant hemisphere. The ictal and postictal aphasia lends confirmation to this.

The first patient had an aura with each occurrence of left temporal lobe spiking discharge. This was documented on audiovisual tape recording by having the patient signal to indicate the point in the music at which the aura of numbness and tingling and the *deja vu* phenomenon occurred. He invariably signalled within one-half second after the appearance of the left anterior temporal spiking discharge. On the few occasions when he had spiking discharges from the right temporal lobe, there was no aura, he did not signal, and none of these discharges proceeded into a seizure. Cases 2 and 3 had no aura with the single spiking discharges. Cases 4 and 5 had no spiking discharges without clinical seizures.

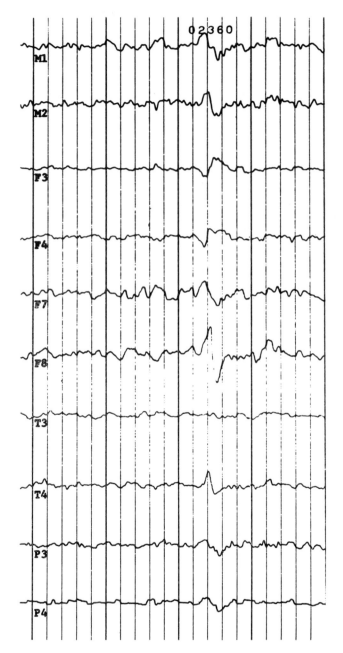

Figure 19. Musicogenic epilepsy. Case 1. Example rare in this patient of right anterior temporal dysrhythmia evoked by music. This never proceeded to clinical seizure, and patient had no aura with the right temporal spiking dysrhythmia.

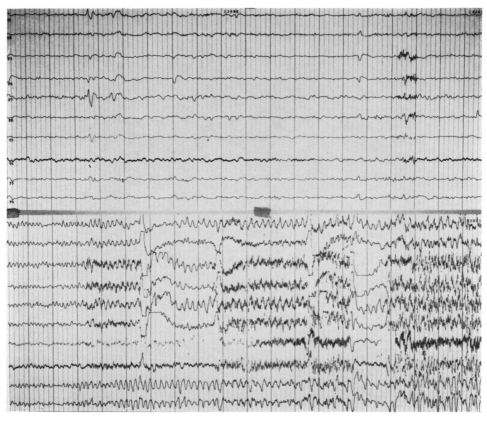

Figure 20. Musicogenic epilepsy. Case 1. Dysrhythmia evoked by music at (F7) left anterior temporal lead (fourth second of recording). Note delay in development of generalized dysrhythmia. Clinical seizure occurred only with delayed development of spread of seizure discharge.

In the first and third patients, polygraphic studies of autonomic variables were performed and showed an alteration in the Galvanic Skin Response (GSR) with each occurrence of a spiking discharge, whether or not it proceeded into a seizure. In the first patient, this might be attributed to his awareness, by means of the occurrence of the aura, of the possibility of an impending seizure. However, in Case 3 (Fig. 21) no auras occurred, and she was entirely unaware of the occurrence of the spiking dysrhythmia. Polygraph studies were not carried out on the other patients.

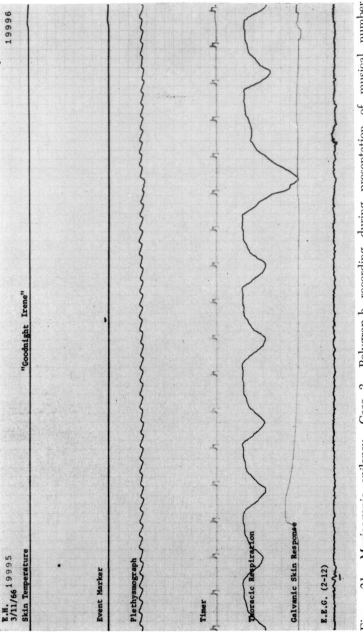

Figure 21. Musicogenic epilepsy. Case 3. Polygraph recording during presentation of musical number ("Goodnight Irene"). Bottom channel is EEG. Small spiking dysrhythmia at right anterior temporal lead is underlined. Galvanic skin response shows change occurring after the temporal evoked spike. Patient had no aura with this dysrhythmia.

It is not necessary for the patients to concentrate upon the music. Seizures may be evoked by the appropriate music while the patient is engaged in conversation or reading for comprehension. As noted above, Case 1 had a seizure while performing his morning ablutions when a patient in a distant room had his radio playing the evoking music softly. The patient was unaware of this. Therefore, the intensity of the stimulus in musicogenic epilepsy is not an important factor. It appears that any stimulus strength adequate to produce a response in the temporal lobe is adequate to evoke a dysrhythmia or seizure. This is unlike the situation in visually induced epilepsy or startle-acousticomotor epilepsy where stimulus intensity is a definite factor.

Moreover, in musicogenic epilepsy the seizure response can be elicited by monaural stimulation even when the decibel level is kept below 60 decibels (Fig. 22). It was noted in Chapter 3 in the discussion of acousticomotor epilepsy, that monaural stimulations above that level (60 decibels) become binaural by bone conduction, and that monaural stimulations in acousticomotor epilepsy below that level do not evoke seizures. In musicogenic epilepsy, however, monaural stimulations evoke seizures. The decibel level was carefully measured throughout recordings of evoking music, and the level was kept below 60 decibels; the result was that when evoking music was presented to the patient monaurally, seizures occurred. Moreover the simultaneous playing of a particular musical number previously shown not to evoke seizures into the other ear did not prevent the occurrence of the seizure, thus suggesting a discriminating ability of the epileptogenic cortex to ascertain the occurrence of the specific, noxious, musical number.

The peculiar discriminative nature of the epileptogenic focus in this form of reflex epilepsy is further indicated by the following study. In Case 1, when one melody which evoked seizures was "scrambled" with two other musical numbers which did not evoke seizures and the conglomerate was played binaurally, the epileptogenic focus determined the presence of the noxious musical number and responded by inducing a seizure.

In two of the patients, the first and third, during medication-induced sleep, seizures were evoked by playing music which

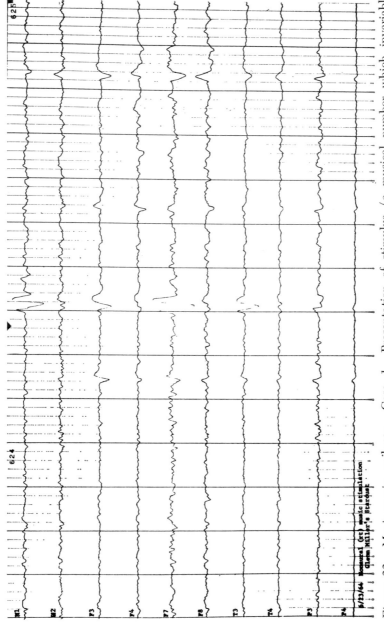

Figure 22. Musicogenic epilepsy. Case 1. Presentation of stimulus (a musical number which invariably evoked seizures or dysrhythmia) to one ear only, by means of stereo earphones. Spiking dysrhythmia evoked from left anterior temporal region (F7) within eight seconds of presentation. Each dark vertical line represents one second.

had evoked seizures in the waking state. In Case 5, during sleep, music evoked an electrical seizure without a clinical component. Hoheisel[12] also observed the induction of seizures during sleep. Many of these patients have nocturnal seizures and this, coupled with the role of memory factors in musicogenic epilepsy, leads to the speculation that the nocturnal seizures might result from the dreaming of music.

Inevitably in a condition as complex as musicogenic epilepsy, the possible role of emotional factors is introduced, especially since music arouses emotional and autonomic responses.[17, 19] However, other authors deny this.[18] In view of the EEG findings in the well-documented cases, there can be no doubt that musicogenic epilepsy is due to an organic cause. But the role of emotional factors is difficult to ascertain. The five cases in the study showed a wide variation of attitudes. The first and third patients went to great length to shun music, avoiding theaters, churches, and restaurants where music was played and requesting their physicians and dentist to turn off the music in the office before they arrived. Both of them enjoyed listening to music, but the first patient was frightened when presented in the laboratory with anything even approximating the type of music which evoked his seizures. By contrast, the second patient was quite indifferent. The fourth patient was enamoured of Rock and Roll music despite the fact that seizures occurred when he listened to it. The fifth patient made no attempt to avoid music, even such simple attempts as not listening to the radio when alone.

The patient's emotional reaction to the type of music is unimportant. Seizures may be induced by music which is either pleasant or unpleasant for the patient. For example, the fifth patient had seizures to a music number ("Amos Moses") which she specificially did not like. She had not heard it before, and the rhythm was distasteful. However, she also had seizures to religious hymns of her own denomination and to other music which she liked.

Seizures may be evoked not only by well-known pleasurable music but by pleasurable music which has never been heard before. Our third patient avoided exposure to music for many years after she became aware of the cause of her problem.

After the therapeutic process had proceeded sufficiently, we began to review the music of the intervening era during which she had deliberately avoided music stimulation. She particularly liked the songs of *The Sound of Music,* which she had never heard before. The song "Maria" was especially pleasing to her, and she requested its frequent playing. At that point, her EEG, her GSR, and plethysmographic studies of her digits were being recorded. She showed vasodilation in her fingers (which indicates pleasure), and right temporal evoked EEG spikes with accompanying GSR changes. Music she had never heard before; music she liked with subjective and objective evidence of her pleasure, and yet she was on the verge of a clinical seizure!

In view of the foregoing, emotional factors can play but a small role, if any, in the evocation of musicogenic epilepsy. This is indicated by the definitive electroencephalographic changes evoked, the patients' unawareness of the true nature of the disease for long periods of time after the onset, the possibility of evocation during sleep, and the evocation by pleasurable as well as unpleasureable music and by music never before heard by the patient.

As noted above, the evoking stimulus in the music is usually subtle and lies in the theme of the music rather than in the instrumentation. Reese[19] pointed this out as long ago as 1948, and his findings have since been confirmed by others.[20] However, there are in the literature some patients with musicogenic epilepsy whose seizures were induced by the sounds of a particular instrument,[13, 21] a particular tone of a bell,[7] or even by a siren as well as by radio music.[12] There are therefore probably two types of musicogenic epilepsy: (a) those dependent upon mechanical factors and (b) those evoked by themes.

The electroencephalographic studies both in the Madison laboratory and of the authors quoted have demonstrated a focal epileptogenic abnormality. This abnormality is predominantly temporal lobe in location, usually unilateral, but not necessarily related to the dominant hemisphere as indicated by the studies by Gornik[22] and by Barrios del Risco and Esslen.[20] However, there are studies including the one documented herein which suggest that there is a relationship to cerebral dominance.

Although the discharging lesions are known to be in the temporal lobe, the etiology may vary. A few cases are considered posttraumatic. However, only two cases, including the first study case (who subsequently died of pneumonia), have come to autopsy, and in neither was there a gross or microscopic lesion discernible. This of course is not unusual in temporal lobe epilepsy, as shown by examination of specimens obtained by means of temporal lobectomy for treatment of temporal lobe epilepsy.

Some variation occurs in the type of seizures reported in musicogenic epilepsy. Psychomotor or temporal lobe automatisms are the most common and occurred in all five of the cases studied, but major motor seizures have also been reported. The latter may or may not have a focal onset. The case reported by Titeca[4] is especially interesting, for when the patient heard languid music at home, she had minor motor seizures; if away from home, psychomotor seizures. The temporal lobe seizures may be mild and only *deja vu* in type. Some authors report petit mal seizures, but one wonders if these were not really temporal lobe "absences." In the Study Case 3, at age ten when playing the organ at church, she would stop, stare, "black out," and have to be carried out. The seizures gradually became more complex, and the pattern changed to typical temporal lobe automatisms.

The natural history of this affliction is, understandably, not known. The cases are too few, the manifestations varied, and the cause obscure. Administration of anticonvulsant medications rarely satisfactorily alleviates the condition. The medications may prevent generalized motor seizures but do not affect the incidence of the evoked temporal lobe seizures. The report of the development over the years of cerebellar ataxia in patients on anticonvulsant medication[4] suggests that this may be the result of medication rather than the disease. One author[4] reports an attenuation of musicogenic epilepsy after ten years, during which the patient listened to no music.

Many authors feel that this illness is not too important, that the patient need only to avoid music. Unfortunately, the technical development of transistor and battery-operated radios, the widespread use of car radios, and the commercially piped-in music cause a severe limitation of activities. Both of our male patients lost their positions because of seizures occurring at work. All five patients suffered embarrassment because of seizures evoked in church, airports, or other public places.

REFERENCES

1. Forster, F. M.: Reading epilepsy, musicogenic epilepsy and allied disorders. In Myklebust, H.: *Prog. in Learning Disorders,* 3rd ed. New York, Grune, 1975.
2. Merzheevski, I. P.: Sloochai epilepsi pripedki kotorsi vizibayootsya nekotopemi musikelnimi tonomi. Minutes Meeting, S *Petersburg Soc Psychiat,* 1884.
3. Critchley, M.: Musicogenic epilepsy. *Brain, 60:*13, 1937.
4. Titeca, J.: L'epilepsie musicogenique. Revue general à propos d'un cas personnel suivi pendant quatorze ans. *Acta Neurol Belg, 65:*598, 1965.
5. Weber, R.: Musikogene epilepsie. *Nervenarzt, 27:*337, 1956.
6. Joynt, J., Green, D., and Green, R.: Musicogenic epilepsy, *JAMA, 179:*125, 1962.
7. Poskanzer, C., Brown, E., and Miller, H.: Musicogenic epilepsy caused only by a discrete frequency band of church bells. *Brain, 85:*77, 1962.
8. Pascher, W. and Rollin, H.: Akustiche Reflex epilepsien. *Nervenarzt, 41:*68, 1970.
9. Vercelleto, P.: À propos d'un cas d'epilepsie musicogenique; presentation d'une crise temporale, discussion sur son pont de depart. *Rev Neurol, 88:*379, 1953.
10. Stubbe-Tegelbjaerg, H. P.: On musicogenic epilepsy. *Acta Psychiatr Belg, 24:*679, 1949.
11. Shaw, D. and Hill, D.: A case of musicogenic epilepsy. *J Neurol Neurosurgy and Psychiatry, 10:*107, 1947.
12. Hoheisel, H. P. and Walch, R.: Ein fall von akusticher reflex nepilepsie. *Psychiatr Neurol Med Psychol* (Leipz), 5:194-200, 1953.
13. Strang, R. R.: A case of musical epilepsy. *J Ir Med Assoc, 59:*85, 1966.
14. Piotrokowski, A.: A case of musicogenic epilepsy observed by clinical and bioelectrical methods. *Neurol Neurochir Pol, 9:*39, 1959.
15. Lennox, W. G. and Lennox, M. A.: *Epilepsy and Related Disorders.* 1:265, Boston, Little, 1960.
16. Reifenberg, E.: Beitrag zur kasuistik der musikogenen epilepsie. *Psychiatr Neurol Med Psychol* (Leipz), *10:*88, 1958.

17. Kranidiotis, P. T., Mikropoulos, C. E., and Terendios, E. N.: Remarks on the so-called musicogenic epilepsy. *Acta Neurol Psychiat,* 9:273, 1970.

18. Chrast, B., Kalab, Z., and Skalnik, J.: Observations on musicogenic epilepsy. *Cs Neurol* (Czech), 25:50, 1962.

19. Reese, H. H.: The relation of music to disease of the brain. *Occup Ther,* 27:12, 1948.

20. Barrios del Risco, P. and Esslen, E.: Epilepsia musicogena. *Acta Neurol Lat Am,* 4:130, 1958.

21. Hasaerts, R. and Titeca, J.: Syndrome cerebelleux d'appartion recente dans un cas d'epilepsie musicogenique. *Ann Med Psychol,* 1:555, 1958.

22. Gornik, V. M.: Musicogenic epilepsy. *Zh Nevropatol Osikhiat* (Korsakow), 64:1227, 1964.

CHAPTER 5

EPILEPSY EVOKED BY HIGHER COGNITIVE FUNCTION; COMMUNICATION-EVOKED EPILEPSY (LANGUAGE EPILEPSY: READING EPILEPSY)

THE PUBLICATIONS BY Bickford,[1, 2] in 1954 and 1956, focused attention upon reading epilepsy. Bickford at first divided the cases into primary and secondary reading epilepsy. Those patients whose seizures occurred only with reading were considered primary. Those patients who had seizures at other times and also had seizures when reading were considered secondary.

Since Bickford's original paper, attention has been focused for the most part on the patients considered to have primary reading epilepsy, and approximately forty-eight cases of this entity have been reported. The incidence of diagnosed reading epilepsy would therefore seem to be relatively small. However, since the diagnosis is usually made on the basis of a major motor seizure, and since the minor seizures are not usually appreciated as a seizure manifestation, there are probably a considerable number of cases that have not been brought to medical attention.

The clinical characteristics of the minor seizures evoked by reading are a myoclonic jaw jerk, often with vocalization and frequently with a very transient loss of consciousness; thus the patient may lose his place in the text. This is associated with an EEG dysrhythmia.

The concept has been greatly broadened by the observations of Geschwind and Sherwin,[3] who introduced the concept of language-induced epilepsy, pointing out that patients may have their seizures with language functions other than simple reading, for example, when writing. In view of the results described below, this broadening concept seems entirely appropriate, and reading or language epilepsy should be considered a disorder of communication.

The University of Wisconsin study included fifteen patients with reading epilepsy. Four of these were excluded from the series presented here. Two were excluded because of the infrequency and unpredictability of clinical EEG changes while reading. One of these patients (the first reading epileptic the author was able to study), was a thirty-two-year-old female, Air Force dependent at Tachikawa United States Air Force Base, Japan. She had a history of jaw jerking while reading, and while the author was consulting at the Base in 1966, she read in the EEG laboratory for four hours, and only one temporal lobe spiking discharge occurred. It was not deemed feasible to transport her to the University of Wisconsin on the basis of this infrequent occurrence. Another patient, a male studied at the University of Wisconsin, was not included in the series because of a similar experience, namely the occurrence of a spiking discharge only when he had read for a number of hours.

Two other patients not included in the series in this chapter are discussed in Chapter 15. They had managed to control the disease by avoidance of reading over a period of years. The remaining eleven patients are included in this series. Brief abstracts of their clinical histories follow:

CASE REPORTS

CASE 1. This patient was an eighteen-year-old high school graduate. For twenty months prior to admission, the patient had noted a peculiar nervous feeling while reading aloud. Six months prior to admission, while reading the George Bernard Shaw play *Anthony and Cleopatra*, he stopped and muttered "Ah" several times in several seconds; he also noted at that time "a strange jerking feeling in my face." This happened again six times while reading aloud. The teacher did not call on him again until one month later, and as the patient was again reading aloud he hesitated, kept muttering "Ah"—finally lost consciousness and proceeded to have what his teacher described as a "typical convulsive seizure." Since the major seizure, he had been taking diphenylhydantoin 100 mg three times daily without control of the minor reading-induced seizures, but has had no subsequent major seizures.

The past medical history was not remarkable. The patient finished high school with average grades and was planning a technical course of study for the future. A maternal great uncle had "epilepsy."

The general physical and neurological examinations were within normal limits. Chest X rays and admission laboratory studies, including skull X rays and brain scan, were normal. The routine resting and sleep electroencephalograms were unremarkable. Neuropsychologic test data demonstrated the patient to be functioning currently at the lower end of the average range of intelligence (Full Scale IQ 90) and exhibiting very mild adaptive defiicits. The Minnesota Multiphasic Personality Inventory (MMPI) profile generated by the patient was not suggestive of significant emotional disturbance.

Case 2.   This patient was a twenty-one-year-old, junior student of architectural engineering at the University of Texas. At the age of seventeen, he first noted jaw jerking while reading. He observed that he could avoid this by discontinuing reading. However, after several months, on one occasion the jaw jerking was followed by loss of consciousness, and tonic-clonic movements were reported. This sequence of minor motor seizures progressing to major motor seizures occurred on two other occasions in the intervening period. He felt that both minor and major seizures occurred when he read technical texts and journals and other reading material but not while reading mathematical formulae. Also, the longer he read, the more frequently the minor seizures occurred.

Past medical history included mumps with associated orchitis in 1964. At that time he also had a duodenal ulcer. He had had bronchitis. He was told he had a thyroid deficiency and was put on ½ gr of thyroid a day approximately three years ago. He stated that his basal metabolic rate had been minus 28 percent at that time. Family history was negative for epilepsy. Review of systems was negative. It was noted that he had headaches when he became "nervous," but these were relieved by aspirin.

Physical and neurological examinations were normal. Admission laboratory studies including skull X ray, chest X ray, brain scan and protein-bound iodine (PBI) were all normal.

CASE 3. This patient, a nineteen-year-old, unemployed white male from Milwaukee, terminated school after eleven years (rather unsuccessful years because of his reading epilepsy). He had been extremely difficult to persuade to come to Madison. He was reluctant to leave Milwaukee because "Madison is too far" and refused to stay overnight, thus truncating the laboratory studies.

He had rheumatic fever at some time during his childhood, and had received a head injury at age nine. The injury consisted of a concussion, after which he had difficulty focusing his eyes and was admitted to St. Mary's Hospital in Milwaukee. At the age of eleven, he noticed that he had jaw jerks when he was reading. These progressed to major motor seizures on four occasions. He was taking diphenylhydantoin 50 mg three times a day and mepharbital 100 mg twice a day at the time of study.

General physical and neurological examinations were normal. Detailed laboratory studies were not possible to obtain because of his poor cooperation.

CASE 4. This patient was a seventeen-year-old, male, high school junior. He was previously reported by Bennett et al.,[5] and the author had the opportunity to participate in his work-up at the University of Utah. He was apparently unaffected by epilepsy until about the age of twelve when he had his first seizure, characterized by stiffening of the jaw with tonic-clonic spasms, while reading a book. This was followed by a "hot" sensation in the low back and epigastrium, and then by loss of consciousness. There were no witnesses, and he was unaware whether he had generalized spasms. On awakening, he was on the floor and felt extremely fatigued. This was followed by a postictal bitemporal headache which lasted for the rest of the day.

The next seizure, at age thirteen, was identical to the first one and was likewise precipitated by reading. In the interim and up to the present, he has continued to have seizures, occurring mostly when he has been reading for some time and characterized by jaw jerking; if he stopped reading this would abate spontaneously. A month after the first seizure he was placed on Dilantin therapy 100 mg three times a day.

The past history revealed the usual childhood illnesses. At the age of seven, the patient sustained a depressed skull fracture of the left frontal region and was operated upon for this. At age fourteen he fell down a hill on his bicycle, with questionable head injury and loss of consciousness.

Family history revealed the mother to have seizures similar to the son's provoked by reading, starting at the age of sixteen. At age forty, an aunt had seizures, but not provoked by reading. A younger aunt, age thirty-two, has had grand mal seizures since the age of two. An aunt of the paternal grandfather and three of the patient's siblings are also reported to have seizures.

Physical and neurological examinations were negative.

Laboratory data were normal. Neuropsychological testing revealed a Full Scale IQ of 94, Verbal 95, and Performance 92. There was no evidence of focal cerebral involvement on neuropsychological tests at the University of Utah. The patient was left handed, left eyed and right footed, but did strum a guitar and throw with his right hand. His skull X rays were negative except for the evidence of the previous surgical procedure. Resting and sleep EEGs were normal. Hyperventilation and photic stimulation responses were also normal.

CASE 5. The patient was a thirty-six-year-old, housewife, mother, and former secretary. At the age of sixteen, while riding on a school bus and reading, she had her first convulsion. She realized that for some time prior to that she had had jaw jerks when reading, but did not understand the significance until they culminated in a convulsive seizure. She has had approximately six major motor seizures while reading, each preceded by the minor seizures. She had only one major motor seizure when not reading. This was sixteen years ago while in the hospital at the time of the delivery of her first child.

Phenobarbital and diphenylhydantoin had been prescribed for her, but she was very irregular in taking these medications. She has not taken them in the past thirteen years, except immediately before one of her deliveries when she would again reinstitute medication. She has seven children.

The family history reveals that she was fifth in birth order. Her brother, who was second in birth order, had seizures when reading. Another brother, who is fourth in birth order, had seizures, but these were not apparently related to reading.

As far as she knows, her birth and delivery were normal. She is said to have had scarlet fever, with a "relapse" at the age of four or five. At the age of thirteen, she was thrown from a horse and was dazed and had headaches for sometime afterwards.

Physical and neurological examinations were entirely normal. Laboratory tests were normal.

CASE 6. The patient was a seventeen-year-old, male high school student. For the past three years, he was aware of the occurrence of involuntary movements of his jaw. These occurred only while reading and usually while reading aloud. The patient had no other associated symptoms, but the jaw jerks tended to occur almost every time he read in class. Approximately two years prior to admission, the patient had a similar episode while reading at home, followed by a tonic seizure after which the patient was amnestic for approximately one hour. He was placed on diphenylhydantoin and at the time of the study was taking 300 mg per day.

Past medical history and review of systems were unremarkable. The family history revealed that his maternal grandmother had grand mal seizures.

Physical and neurological examinations were normal. Neuropsychological testing was entirely within normal limits, with a Full Scale IQ of 118, Verbal of 117, and Performance IQ of 116 The Wide Range Achievement Test was consistent with grade placement and IQ. No tests of adaptive abilities yielded results in the impaired range. Motor and sensory testing was within normal limits.

CASES 7 AND 8. These patients were identical twins, age twenty-nine, both housewives, both of whom finished high school and stopped school at that point because of reading epilepsy. Both were the product of an uneventful pregnancy other than precipitous delivery. Each had a normal childhood and received excellent grades in school.

Both sisters, somewhere near the age of sixteen, began to have clonic jaw movements with brief loss of consciousness, but no postictal state. These seizures occurred whether they were reading aloud or silently. Neither of them ever had a definite major seizure, although by self-report, patient 8 on one occasion became unconscious and slumped to the floor. There was no witness to this event. In retrospect, she probably had a major seizure but this cannot be confirmed.

Because of the peculiar affinity of twins for each other, one of them confided to the other that she had for some months been having something unusual happen to her while she read. The other twin then stated she too was having similar occurrences. Presumably both of them had had this experience for several months, so the age of onset may have been relatively close, although this is conjectural. They tested each other by observing one another read and brought the evoked minor seizures to the attention of their parents. They were diagnosed as having reading epilepsy by their physician and subsequently referred to the University of Wisconsin.

In addition to the jaw jerking while reading, each of the twins had some difficulty when writing. The same sequence happened except instead of the jaw jerk, their hands "froze," and they were unable to use them for a few seconds. One of the sisters plays the piano and may have the same clonic jerk or freezing of the hand while playing the piano. An attempt was made by one of the twins (Case 8), to learn Braille from a friend. This was with the intent of being able to go on to college and following her course work by reading Braille. However, when she became proficient in this, seizures occurred when reading Braille. These seizures involved the hand rather than the jaw.

The past medical histories were noncontributory. One of the twins was in an automobile accident with cervical spine injury, but this was after the onset of the reading epilepsy. There was no other family history of seizures. Both patients' physical and neurological examinations were negative.

Neuropsychological reports on the twins showed a marked similarity. Both were in the high-average range of intellectual functioning. Their motor and sensory performances were excellent.

The identical nature of their twinhood was so striking that we found it necessary to have them dress in a conspicuously different manner while in the laboratory so that their AV tapes could be identified. Detailed studies of finger whorls, ear configuration and blood typings[9] indeed confirmed that they were identical twins.

CASE 9. This patient is also discussed in Chapter 6. The patient was a thirty-one-year-old married accountant. At the age of fourteen years, he suffered a football head injury, without loss of consciousness, and was amnesic for about three hours. Approximately one month later, he had a seizure which was characterized by sudden loss of consciousness for ten minutes. No postictal phenomena was observed. Apparently there were no tonic-clonic movements. Over the next several years, he had eight of these seizures, and two years after, up until the age of nineteen years, he had occasional flinging of his arms with loss of consciousness but not falling to the floor. With none of these were tonic-clonic movements observed. He did bite his tongue on several occasions, but was never incontinent. Postictal tiredness, confusion, etc. were not reported. Shortly after the seizures began, he was started on diphenylhydantoin 100 mg twice a day. No EEG was taken. The patient had not taken his medication faithfully.

He noted when studying or reading aloud, especially if reading quickly, that he would suddenly stop reading and say a few garbled words for a matter of seconds. No loss of consciousness occurred with these episodes, and they never progressed into a major motor seizure. Upon detailed questioning, it appeared that most if not all of the major seizures occurred while he was playing cards and concentrating on the "hand" dealt to him. For these reasons he is also considered in Chapter 6.

There was a family history of seizures. His mother sustained a head injury in her teens and had approximately five years of seizures which were never treated, and apparently were self-limited. The patient and his mother have otosclerosis. He has one child, seven years old, who has minimal brain dysfunction, recently has become night-blind, and is now being evaluated for the possibility of retinitis pigmentosa.

Physical and neurological examinations were normal.

CASE 10. This sixteen-year-old, right handed, male high

school sophomore was admitted with a history of a seizure episode four days prior to admission. While he was reading the sports section of the newspaper, his mother found the patient with arms outstretched and hands clasped. The neck was hyperextended and the legs were stiff, with rhythmic jerking movements of all extremities. This was accompanied by moaning and cyanosis. No incontinence or tongue biting was noted. The episode lasted approximately one to two minutes, followed by several minutes of thrashing about on the floor, eyes open but unresponsive. The entire episode lasted approximately ten to twenty minutes, with the patient becoming aware of his surroundings while in the ambulance. The patient was amnesic for the event and experienced mild malaise for several hours.

There was a history of approximately one year's duration of facial twitching when the patient was reading, especially if he had to read aloud. He could not articulate adequately when this occurred, and the episode usually lasted less than one minute.

A positive family history of epilepsy was reported with a maternal cousin having recently experienced a single generalized seizure.

There was no history of significant head trauma or serious illness. Upon admission, he was receiving diphenylhydantoin 300 mg per day and phenobarbital 120 mg per day.

Physical and neurological examinations were normal, as were routine laboratory studies.

CASE 11. This patient was a twenty-five-year-old housewife and was the maternal first cousin of Case 10. For approximately four and one-half years, she had noticed when reading aloud, jerking of her jaw and some slurring of speech. After some three years of these minor seizures (which were not recognized as such), when reading, she cried out to her husband, who noted she had some jaw jerking. She then lost consciousness, became cyanotic, and had a generalized tonic-clonic seizure with postictal drowsiness. Following this, she was begun on diphenylhydantoin 300 mg a day and had no further major seizures, but the minor attacks evoked by reading continued.

Past history was potentially significant in that she had meningitis at about the age of four, with a residual deafness of the right ear.

Physical and neurological examinations were normal with the exception of the hearing loss in the right ear.

Laboratory studies, including EEG in the resting state, during hyperventilation, and with visual stimulation, were normal.

CLINICAL FEATURES

The salient clinical features of the eleven patients studied in this series are presented in Table VIII. The ratio of male to female (7:4) is inconclusive, although this entity may be more common in males. The age at time of study is highly variable, but the age of onset is indeed significant—the onset in all our patients (except Case 11, at age twenty) was in the teens; this is in accord with the literature. Chen and Little[6] reported the oldest age of onset (age thirty-six).

There was an exceptionally high incidence of seizures in the families of the patients reported here. Seven of the nine families have a history of epilepsy, and in four of the families there is a history of reading epilepsy. This strongly suggests the possibility of an hereditary factor. This has been previously commented upon by Rowan et al.[7] and by Matthews and Wright,[8] each of whom reported a mother and daughter with the condition. These authors suggested that reading epilepsy might well be hereditary and due to a dominant gene.

The occurrence in Cases 7 and 8, confirmed in the laboratory, of reading epilepsy in identical twins strongly suggested the possibility of an hereditary factor in at least some cases of reading epilepsy.[9] The monozygocity of our twins was established not only by their identical appearance, but also by their fingerprint conformations and blood types. They and their parents and siblings were studied for twenty-three blood types, and the twins were found to be identical in these regards and different from other members of the family. Since there was no history of seizures in the family other than the twins, no mode of inheritance could be determined.

However, the opportunity to study Cases 10 and 11, first cousins, gave the study team an opportunity to screen the siblings and parents of these patients. In this study,[10] two undetected instances of reading epilepsy were uncovered in the

TABLE VIII

Clinical Data – Reading Epilepsy

Case No.	Age	Sex	Age at Onset	Family History		Other Illness	Occupation	Education	Type of Seizures		Routine EEG	EEG Dys While Reading		Dominance		
				Positive For Epilepsy	Positive For Reading Epilepsy				Minor	Major				Eye	Hand	Foot
1	17	M	16½	+	0	0	Student	12 yrs.	+	+	N	S/SW	L.A.T.	R	R	?
2	21	M	18	0	0	0	Student	15 yrs.	+	+	N	S	Syl R&L	R	R	R
3	19	M	11	0	0	Rheum fever Head injury	None	11 (drop-out)	+	+	N	S/SW	L.T.	?	R	?
4	17	M	12	+	+	Head injury	None	12 yrs.	+	+	N	S/SW	RPC&C	L	L	L
5	35	F	16	+	+	Head injury	H. W. & Secy	12 yrs.	+	+	N	S	RC	?	R	?
6	17	M	14	+	0	0	Student	11 yrs.	+	+	N	S	Vertex L.T.	R	R	R
7	29	F	16	+	+ Identical	0	H.W.	12 yrs.	+	0	N	S/SW	L.F.T.	R	R	R
8	29	F	16	+	+ Twins	0	H.W.	12 yrs.	+	?	N	S/SW	L.F.T.	R	R	R
9	31	M	13	+	0	Otosclerosis	Accountant	16 yrs.	+	+	N	S	Vertex (C.Z.) bifrontal	R	R	R
10	16	M	15	+	+	0	Student	10 yrs.	+	+	N	S	L.F.T.	R	R	R
11	25	F	21	+	+	Post-meningitis	H.W.	10 yrs.	+	+	N	S	L.A.T.	R	R	R

siblings of Case 10. These studies confirmed that the hereditary factor plays an important role in reading epilepsy and is on the basis of a dominant gene with a low penetrance. Moreover, this suggests that reading epilepsy is more prevalent than suspected, since in the main, only cases with major motor seizures have been discovered.

In the study material, as in the reported cases in the literature,[11-13, 30] there was no statistically significant predominant etiology present. Three of the patients had received head injuries. Two of these were mild concussions, and one patient had had a compound fracture of the frontal area. One patient had had meningitis. There were no other significant medical conditions in the past or present histories.

As might be expected in this age group, four of the patients were students. Of the older patients, two (the twins) had finished high school and had not proceeded to college because of the reading epilepsy. One patient (Case 3) had dropped out of high school because of the seizures. Reading epilepsy is therefore a serious deterrent to education.

Reading epilepsy is usually not recognized as such until major motor seizures develop. As in the reported cases in the literature, nine and possibly ten of the patients in the study had major motor seizures when they continued to read after the repeated occurrence of minor seizures.

The characteristic minor seizures in reading epilepsy, as noted before, consist of a break in reading, jaw or jaw and tongue myoclonic jerk, with vocalization as a loud "Ah" or even a sibilant hiss. The vocalization and the jaw jerk, however, occurred only when reading aloud. When reading quietly, no motor manifestation was visible, but the patients were aware of the subjective sensation of the seizures. When requested, they would signal the occurrence of this clinical subjective manifestation. There was a close correlation between the appearance of the dysrhythmia in the EEG and either the clinically observed seizure or the signal given by the patient indicating they were subjectively aware of the seizure manifestation (Fig. 23). Sometimes a brief lapse of consciousness occurred, as indicated by the patient losing his place in the text. These minor seizures usually lasted less than a second. In Case 10 (Fig. 24),

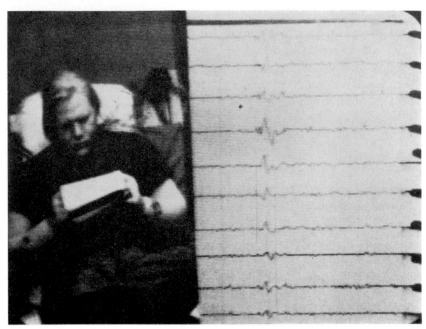

Figure 23.   Reading epilepsy. Case 3. Patient reading meaningful, non-remembered material. EEG dysrhythmia accompanied break in reading. EEG dysrhythmia is primarily left anterior temporal (fourth channel from top) and indicating some spread to other cortical areas.

however, the seizures evoked in the laboratory were often as long as four seconds in duration. This permitted special observations. The patient was aware of an aphasic component, stating that during the seizure he could not talk. It became evident that during the seizures, he was aware of the nature and the name of an object shown him, but was unable to verbally identify it. He could not respond verbally to simple commands such as "are you all right?" until the end of the dysrhythmia but could carry out such nonverbal commands as "close your eyes."

The major motor seizures apparently have no unusual manifestation except that they occur in the course of reading and following the appearance of a number of minor seizures. None of the patients studied experienced a major motor seizure, even though the patients were recorded and studied for as long as four hours per day over a two-week period. However, no attempts were made to precipitate a major seizure by prolonged

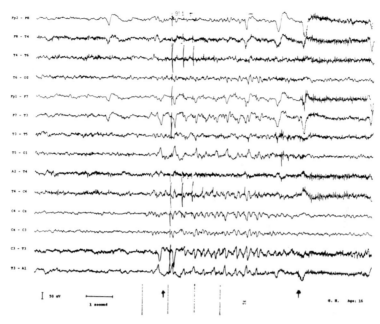

Figure 24. Reading epilepsy. EEG in Case 10 showing prolonged dysrhythmia. This was associated with aphasia. Primary EEG dysrhythmia was in the presumed dominant hemisphere (left) and in the frontotemporal region.

reading with many repeated minor seizures. Critchley et al.[14] witnessed a major motor seizure in one of their patients, and the seizure was focal in onset beginning with head deviation to the right.

In all of the laboratory patients except Case 10, the resting and sleep EEGs were normal. In this patient, two types of dysrhythmia occurred. A generalized slow wave dysrhythmia occurred without clinical counterparts and was seen in sensory deprivation, sleep, and during various activities. This was not reproducible; for example, it occurred the first time that mathematical computations were administered, but on repeated trials over three days, mathematical problems of the same type and of differing types failed to evoke this dysrhythmia. During reading, however, a significant, left temporal frontal spiking dysrhythmia occurred and was accompanied by clinical seizures.

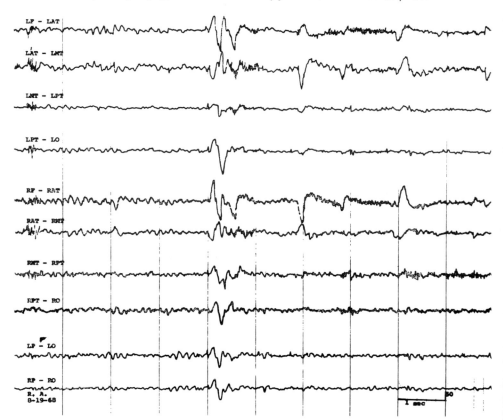

Figure 25. Reading epilepsy. EEG in Case 1 when reading non-memorized, meaningful material. Evoked dysrhythmia appears generalized but begins in left temporal region (See also Figure 73). Reprinted from *Neurology* © 1969 by The New York Times Media Company, Inc.

In all patients during reading, paroxysmal discharges occurred, either spiking or spike and slow wave in type (Fig. 25). The location of the dysrhythmia varied from patient to patient, from frontal to temporal to central foci, with some mixtures. It should be noted that in no patient was the dysrhythmia primarily recorded from the posterior or occipital portion but always from the anterior portion of the brain.

The laterality of the dysrhythmia is especially significant when compared with the cerebral dominance. In none of the patients was the intracarotid amytal test employed for the determination of cerebral dominance. The risks of the test were not justifiable since none of the patients were being considered for surgical therapy. Hand, eye, and foot preferences were determined in testing in the neuropsychology laboratory in eight of the patients, and handedness by performance in the research laboratory in the remaining three patients. In eight patients the EEG focus was in the presumed dominant hemisphere, in two patients the dysrhythmia was bilateral, and in only one patient was the dysrhythmia evoked in the presumed non-dominant hemisphere. This strongly suggests that reading epilepsy is a manifestation of disorder in the dominant hemisphere.

The general physical and neurological examinations were normal. No abnormalities were detected by skull roentgenography or brain scan. Cases 3 and 5 did not have these latter tests. None of the patients were retarded and they varied from low-normal to a Full Scale Wechsler Adult Intelligence Scale (WAIS) IQ of 118.

Various theories have been proposed to explain the evocation of seizures by reading. These theories include proprioceptive feedback from the extraocular movements or from the muscles involved in vocalization, especially those of the jaw, the printed page serving as a pattern stimulus, the role of concentration upon the printed material, and the nature of the material as it applies to the particular patient. Eye strain, sleep deprivation, fasting, and fatigue[24] have been assigned contributory roles.

In order to test these hypotheses, the patients were subjected to the following standard test battery.

STANDARD TESTING OF PATIENTS WITH READING EPILEPSY

To study the role of the possible pathophysiological mechanisms noted above, it was considered necessary to impose a uniform procedure to the study of patients with reading epilepsy. Therefore, the standard battery described here was devised.

All patients were presented first with meaningful, non-memorized reading material. This included a popular magazine which was easily read and of general interest, plus parts of a play (George Bernard Shaw's *Anthony and Cleopatra*) which was more difficult to read. The latter was presented not only in the horizontal type as published but also in a vertical format, one word on a line, and also one letter on a line. It was read therefore from top to bottom to test the effect of vertical reading.

The patients were also presented with reading material which was well known to them and was at least partially memorized: the Psalms of the Old Testament, (twenty-second, twenty-third, and twenty-fourth were used) and also the New Testament, Matthew Chapter 6, Verses 5 to 19. Both the King James and the Douay version were available in the laboratory. Since all of our patients were Christians, it was not necessary to introduce the Koran or the Talmud, and of course the Psalms could be used for Jewish patients. This choice of religious literature was made because parts of these passages are almost universally known and include not only such frequently read or spoken parts as the twenty-third Psalm and the Lord's Prayer but also less familiar parts, such as for example, the twenty-second and twenty-fourth Psalms and the sections of Matthew preceding and following the Lord's Prayer.

The patients were also given columns of digits to read both vertically and horizontally and were presented with complex mathematical problems requiring either division or multiplication.

The foreign language presentations were not standardized because the choice of language depended upon the patient's lack of facility in the language to be selected. Care was taken to avoid any effect of a learned language; for example, if the patient had studied Latin, Romance languages were not used, but instead, German was selected.

The patients were tested while reading aloud, reading quietly with lip and tongue movement and reading quietly without obvious movement of lip or tongue. Patients were also tested reading with the vision of one eye occluded to permit study of monocular presentations of the stimulus material.

Each patient was presented with a playback of the audio portion of the AV tape, thus enabling him to hear the sounds of his voice as he read the various passages, including those in which he had had seizures. During this, he was observed for possible occurrence of seizures or EEG dysrhythmia.

RESULTS OF TESTING

Table IX presents the results of applying this battery of tests to the study series of patients. The testing was begun with meaningful, nonfamiliar material. The length of time the patient had to read in order to evoke a seizure in the laboratory is noted in the first column. The length of time varied with each presentation of reading material, and the longest time for a given patient was the very first presentation. The length of time varied in these eleven patients between one and forty minutes. The time may be much longer of course, as has been noted earlier in this chapter, for patients excluded from the study.

All of the patients had seizures when reading the meaningful material which they had not committed to memory and which was unfamiliar. For familiar material, the patients were presented with something that each knew from memory as described above. This test was not in the battery at the time of studying the first patient, hence the question mark in the column. Of the remaining ten patients only one, Case 4, had seizures on reading his version of the Lord's Prayer. In Case 6, a Roman Catholic, after he had been shown repeatedly to have no seizures to his version of the Lord's Prayer, a substitution was made of "transubstantial" for "daily" bread. When he blithely arrived at the passage "Give us . . ." he had a seizure as he scanned ahead and found the unusual word (Fig. 26).

In only two patients did reading a foreign language fail to evoke seizures. However, on reviewing the AV tapes at a later date, an explanation was revealed. Neither patient took seriously the matter of a nonunderstood language. Case 2 thought the whole procedure very funny and was laughing throughout the reading of Latin and Spanish. Case 3 was sullen, hostile, and uncooperative and paid little attention to the German. Thereafter each succeeding patient was exhorted to "get something"—whatever he/she could—out of the material; they did try, and they had seizures (Fig. 27). Case 2 was not available for restudy because of distance and occupation, and Case 3 would not return for further study to check this point. Cases 2 and 3 demonstrate that it is not sufficient merely to present nonmeaningful material, but that the patient must be persuaded to try to acquire some knowledge from it.

TABLE IX

RESULTS OF APPLYING STANDARD BATTERY TO PATIENTS WITH READING EPILEPSY

Case No.	Duration Reading	Reading Material		Material Memorized	Reading Digits	Computations	Reading		Direction Reading		Method of Reading			Rehearing
		Meaningful	Non-meaningful				Binoc	Monoc	Horiz	Vert	Silent	Silent with Movement	Aloud	
1	8-12'	+	+	?	+	0	+	+	+	+	0	+	+	0
2	5-10'	+	0	0	0	0	+	+	+	+	+	+	+	0
3	3-10'	+	0	0	0	0	+	+	+	+	+	+	+	0
4	1-15'	+	+	+	+	0	+	+	+	+	+	+	+	0
5	2-5'	+	+	+	0	0	+	+	+	+	+	+	+	0
6	2-19'	+	+	0	+	0	+	+	+	+	+	+	+	0
7	1-5'	÷	+	0	+	0	+	+	+	+	+	+	+	0
8	4-40'	+	+ (by history)	0	+	0	+	+	+	+	+	+	+	0
9	1-7½'	+	+	0	0	0	+	+	+	+	0	+	+	0
10	3-10'	+	+	0	+	0	+	+	+	+	+	+	+	0
11	10"-7'	+	+	0	+	0	+	+	+	+	+	+	+	0

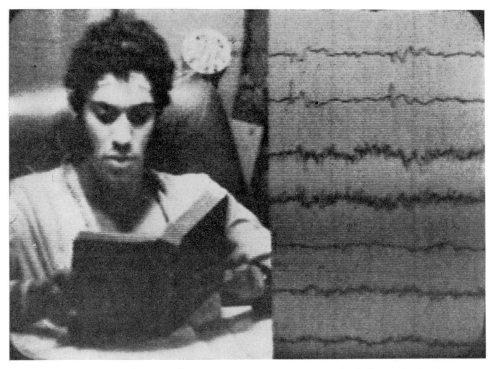

Figure 26. Reading epilepsy. Case 6. Seizure evoked by substitution of unfamiliar word for familiar word in memorized material. EEG dysrhythmia most prominent in left temporal region (third channel from top).

All eleven patients had seizures readily evoked by reading aloud, and all but two of the patients also had seizures when reading quietly, without evidence of movement of the organs of vocalization.

When reading digits, six patients had seizures and five did not. One of the latter (Case 8) had a history of seizures evoked by reading numbers. In retrospect, this failure of digits to evoke seizures is probably due to a testing error. It did not become apparent until working with Case 10 that the digits presented must not be sequential. If they are, the effect is the same as reading memorized material. Prior to that, the testing had sometimes employed sequential numbers. This may well be the reason for the variance obtained.

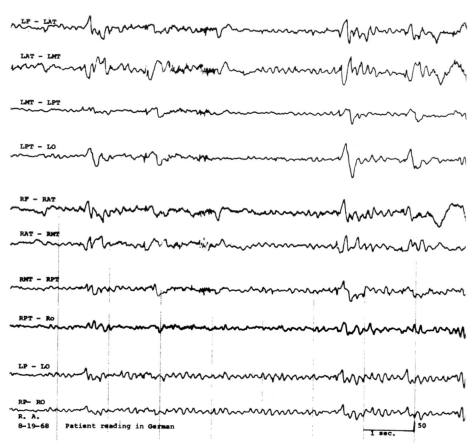

Figure 27.   Reading epilepsy.   Case 1.   EEG dysrhythmia evoked by attempting to obtain information from a nonunderstood foreign language. EEG dysrhythmia is predominently left temporal.   Patient is right handed.

None of the eleven patients had seizures or dysrhythmias evoked by solving mathematical problems.   Both multiplications and divisions were used, usually five or more digits on one part of the problem and three or four on the other.   Therefore, a case similar to that of Ingvarr and Nyman[25] was not encountered in this study, although their patient's seizures may have been evoked by decision making as noted in the following chapter.

The direction of reading had no effect upon the outcome. Reading vertically, one word at a time, evoked seizures as readily as did reading horizontally. Reading one letter at a time in the vertical plane delayed the occurrence of a seizure only until the patient developed a facility in this type of reading.

All eleven patients had seizures evoked when reading monocularly. This was tested for each eye separately to rule out any effect of dominance.

The auditory input of the material read did not evoke seizures or dysrhythmias in any of the patients. No patient had seizures when not reading, but listening to the audioplayback of his own reading which had resulted in seizures. Also, when passages which had evoked seizures were read to the patient by someone else, seizures did not occur. In the case of the twins, having one twin read to the other did not evoke seizures or dysrhythmias in the one who was listening.

The effects of varied illumination levels and of differences in the focus of the printed material were studied in the first several patients in this series. The reading material was projected on a screen with the light intensity of the projector decreased so that the printed matter was barely visible. As soon as it became sufficiently legible, however, seizures were evoked. The material was also presented out of focus and gradually brought into focus. As legibility was attained, seizures again were evoked.

RESULTS OF SPECIAL INDIVIDUALIZED STUDIES

In addition to the standard battery, certain tests were designed for individual patients. Since reading silently did not evoke seizures in Case 1 (previously reported[4]), but reading aloud or with lip movement did, further tests were employed. The patient was studied while humming, whistling, and singing, both from memory and while reading the words. Seizures did not occur in any of these conditions. These tests were carried on for at least as long as the longest period of time necessary to evoke a seizure by reading aloud.

These studies and the concept of reading epilepsy as a communication disorder led to the question, Can reading epilepsy occur when reading Braille? A survey of the Wisconsin School for the Blind revealed no epilectic who might conceivably have reading epilepsy. Case 3, a very cooperative student from the University of Texas, over a weekend during his hospitalization attempted to learn to read Braille under the tutelage of a blind social worker in our hospital. The following Monday, when studied in the laboratory, reading Braille did not evoke a seizure. However he read Braille very slowly and laboriously, and with little facility. This required a great deal of vigilance and was not an adequate test for the hypothesis. However, Case 7 had years ago learned from a blind friend how to read Braille. It was her hope that she might thus be able to go on to college. She found after she developed a facility in reading Braille, seizures occurred. Unfortunately this could not be tested in the laboratory because she had lost her facility for reading Braille over the past six years.

Cases 4, 7, and 8 also had seizures when writing, even when blindfolded. When this occurred, the motor manifestation, rather than being a vocalization, was instead a jerking (clonic) or freezing (tonic) state of the arm or hand (Fig. 28).

Case 7 played piano, and this also evoked a hand jerking or freezing. She was presented with a music score without words, and, on drumming out the treble clef, her right hand "froze." This was associated with the usual EEG dysrhythmia.

Case 4, in addition to seizures on reading and writing, also had occasional seizures on speaking memorized material without reading. This indeed is akin to the case of language epilepsy described by Geschwind and Sherwin.[3] Case 4 has been reported separately by Bennett, Mavor and Jarcho.[5]

Case 5, a secretary, offered some unusual testing opportunities. She took a letter from dictation in shorthand. No dysrhythmia occurred, and there were no seizures while she wrote the shorthand. When, however, she transcribed the shorthand by typing, dysrhythmia occurred (Fig. 29), but only when looking at the shorthand notes—not while looking toward the typewriter. The dysrhythmia was accompanied by hesitation in the typing, but there was no vocalization or jaw jerk. When given a magazine article to type, she did this without difficulty. But when asked to sit back and close her eyes so she could not see the typed material and then tell the physician what she had typed, she

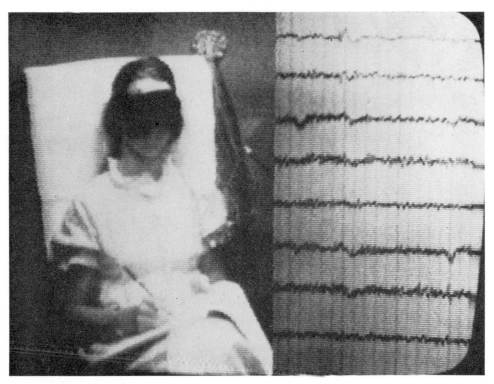

Figure 28. Reading/language epilepsy. Case 7. Seizure evoked by writing, even though blindfolded. Patient's hand "froze" accompanied by EEG dysrhythmia in left frontotemporal region (channels one and two of EEG).

could give little more than the title of the article. Like many secretaries, she had typed the article without making any mental imprint of its contents. When asked to read aloud what she had typed so she could relate information about it later, she had seizures while reading.

She was given a copy of the Koran in Arabic under the impression it was a new kind of shorthand. Staring at it and trying to understand it evoked no seizures, but when she was given the English translation to read, seizures promptly occurred. She volunteered she could not "get anything" out of the Arabic.

Singing was not uniformly employed in the study of these patients. It was, however, tried in all Cases except 3, 5, and 11.

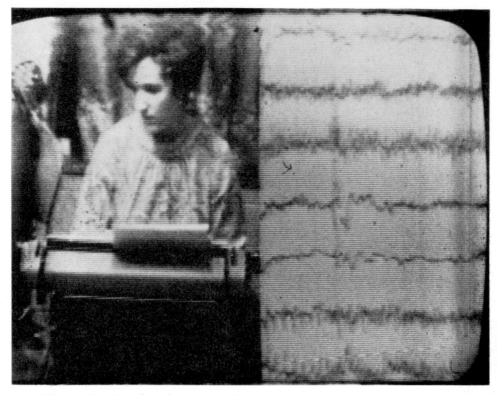

Figure 29.   Reading/language epilepsy. Case 5. Patient is reading short-hand notes and transcribing these. Seizures occur only when patient is looking at notes—not when looking at typewriter. EEG dysrhythmia is most prominent and free of muscle artifact in third chanel from bottom (left anterior temporal). During the occurrence of the dysrhythmia patient's hand "froze" on typewriter.

In Cases 1, 6, and 10, after the patients had had seizures evoked by reading the words of a strange song, they were asked to sing the number to musical accompaniment while reading the words to the song. No seizures occurred. To exclude any memory effect for the protection from seizures in these patients, the process was reversed. The patient sang the new words first without evoking seizures and then read the same words later, causing the seizures to be evoked. Case 4, however, had seizures when singing and in Case 9, seizures occurred with the presentations of unfamiliar songs. For example, when he was given

"Little Town of Bethlehem" to sing, during the first two stanzas there were no difficulties. But during the third and fourth stanzas, seizures occurred. He volunteered that he knew the first two stanzas but did not know the last two. Therefore, for him, the effect of nonmemorized material was the same when singing as when reading.

CONSIDERATIONS OF THE THEORIES IN VIEW OF LABORATORY RESEARCH DATA

A frequently stated theory maintains that the evoking cause of reading epilepsy is the proprioceptive feedback from the extraocular muscles. While this mechanism undoubtedly was at work in the case reported by Alajouanine,[26] this factor is ruled out in the study cases. The occurrence of seizures with changes of direction of eye movement from horizontal to vertical, the failure to evoke seizures by reading memorized material, the occasional absence of seizures when reading nonmeaningful material or digits, and the absence of seizures in computations makes it extremely unlikely that eye movements play a role in the evocation of seizures in most cases of reading epilepsy.

Another theory often stated maintains that the proprioceptive feedback from the muscles of vocalization may represent the evoking stimulus. Admittedly, reading silently without movement of lips was as effective in producing seizures as was reading aloud in nine of the study patients. However, in the first patient, other proprioceptive feedback in humming, whistling, and singing, even while reading the words of the song, did not evoke seizures. Moreover, the feedback from the muscles of vocalization should be no different if the material read is memorized or unfamiliar.

In the cases studied, pattern epilepsy cannot be a factor. The visual pattern is the same for memorized material as it is for new meaningful material. Digits for computation present the same pattern as digits merely to be read. The Arabic script has some similarity to shorthand and yet did not evoke seizures. Also, it should be noted that most patients with pattern epilepsy do not have seizures when viewing patterns monocularly. However, all of the study patients had seizures when reading monocularly. While pattern epilepsy seems to have been the evoking factor in the patient of Mayersdorf and Marshall,[27] this certainly has not played any identifiable role in the study patients.

The concentration of the patient has also been indicated as the evoking cause.[19] This instead should be interpreted as the process of acquisition or dissemination of information. Note the absence of seizures when reading material containing no new information. Concentration itself tends to prevent the seizures. This is indicated by the absence of seizures during mathematical computations, during the laborious reading of Braille, and while reading the words and singing, especially to accompaniment. Indeed, this inhibition by concentration has led to a method of treatment as noted in the chapters on treatment.

However, reading epilepsy is indeed a complex subject. A few of the reported cases obviously have some factors other than communication involved. It is, however, now possible to place the theories in order of importance and to cite opinions and examples of specific cases with different modes of evocation. In their order of importance, the evoking factors appear to be:

1. The process of acquiring or transmitting knowledge, as demonstrated in the patients reported in this chapter.
2. The proprioceptive feedback from extraocular muscles. The case of Alajouanine[26] is an example of this. When the patient followed a light moving in the pattern of the eye movements in reading, seizures occurred.
3. Pattern evocation may play a role in some cases, for example, the two cited by Mayersdorf and Marshall.[27]
4. There is no evidence that feedback from the jaw jerk evokes the seizures. Seizures occur when reading silently. Moreover Bennett et al.[5] showed by simultaneous electromyogram (EMG) and EEG recording that the cortical discharge precedes the jaw jerk.
5. Auditory input, as has been shown, plays no role.

Certain other factors may also play a part. As reported by Critchley, Cobb, and Sears,[14] in some patients the printed material needs to be of a specific printing type and have some personal interest.

It is not surprising that sleep deprivation and fasting may play a role as reported by White.[24] However, these latter cannot be the main neurophysiological factors but only serve as contributory factors.

The motor manifestations in the study patients are of particular interest Objective jaw jerk and vocalization occurred only when reading aloud. No overt clinical manifestations occurred when reading silently, although the patients were subjectively more aware of the occurrence of the dysrhythmia. When the clinical manifestations occurred with a manual communication task such as writing, typing, or playing the piano, the motor manifestation affected the appropriate body part, that is, the upper extremity. This also occurred in the patients reported by Stevens[19] and by Chen and Little.[6] Stevens also noted that when his patient had learned the musical score, reading and playing the piano no longer elicited seizures. This indicated that the learning factor with reference to the musical score served the same purpose as the learning factor did with reading material. Therefore, in communication or language epilepsy, the motor manifestations of seizures depend upon the mode of expression or communication.

In the cases cited here, the process of acquiring or transmitting knowledge by use of language is the most important evoking factor. This concept is supported by the fact that the EEG dysrhythmia in reading epilepsy is primarily in the frontal regions of the brain. Not only is the EEG dysrhythmia anteriorly placed, but from the University of Wisconsin studies, it would seem in most instances to be in the dominant hemisphere. Demonstration of aphasic seizures in reading epilepsy as in Case 10 also suggests that this is a communication disorder. These various facts offer further evidence that reading epilepsy and language epilepsy are not induced by simple visual, proprioceptive, or pattern stimuli but are evoked by higher cognitive functions associated with communication. The communication is not limited to verbal symbols in language but can involve other communications such as musical scores and shorthand symbols, hence the term communication epilepsy. Moreover, the involvement may be in either the afferent or external transmission, or in the efferent or acquisition phases of communication.

REFERENCES

1. Bickford, R. G.: Sensory precipitation of seizures. *J Michigan M Soc,* 53:1018, 1954.
2. Bickford, R. et al.: Reading epilepsy. *Trans Am Neurol Assoc, 81*:100, 1956.
3. Geschwind, N. and Sherwin, I.: Language induced epilepsy. *Arch Neurol, 16*:25, 1967.
4. Forster, F. M., Paulsen, W. A., and Baughman, F. A., Jr.: Clinical therapeutic conditioning in reading epilepsy. *Neurology, 19*:717, 1969.
5. Bennett, D. R., Mavor, H., and Jarcho, L. W.: Language induced epilepsy. Report of a case. *Electroencephalogr Clin Neurophysiol, 30*:159, 1971.
6. Chen, L. T. and Little, S. C.: Reading epilepsy. *Ala J Med Sci,* 8:227, 1971.
7. Rowan, A. J., Heathfield, K. W. G., and Scott, D. F.: Is reading epilepsy inherited? *J Neurol Neurosurg Psychiat, 33*:467, 1970.
8. Matthews, W. and Wright, F.: Hereditary primary reading epilepsy. *Neurology, 17*:919, 1967.
9. Forster, F. M. and Daly, R.: Reading epilepsy in identical twins. *Trans Am Neurol Assoc, 98*:186, 1973.
10. Daly, R. F. and Forster, F. M.: Inheritance of reading epilepsy. *Neurology, 25*:1051, 1975.
11. Zlotow, M.: Primary reading epilepsy. *NY State J Med, 64*:2472, 1964.
12. Tuvo, F., Morandini, N., and Balestra, F.: Sur un nouveau cas d'epilepsie par la lecture. *G psicchiat Neuropat, 94*:155, 1966.
13. Lemmi, H. and Farris, A. A.: Reading epilepsy case report and review of literature. *South Med J, 63*:1431, 1970.
14. Critchley, M. et al.: On reading epilepsy. *Epilepsia, 1*:403, 1959.
15. Norburg, F. and Loeffler, D.: Primary reading epilepsy. *JAMA, 194*: 661, 1963.
16. Bingel, A.: Reading epilepsy. *Neurology, 7*:752, 1957.
17. Lasater, G.: Reading epilepsy. *Arch Neurol, 6*:492, 1962.
18. Baxter, D. and Bailey, A.: Primary reading epilepsy. *Neurology, 11*:445, 1961.
19. Stevens, H.: Reading epilepsy. *N Eng J Med, 257*:165, 1957.
20. Blumenthal, I. and Dunn, A.: Reading epilepsy. *Electroencephalogr Clin Neurophysiol, 14*:270, 1962.
21. Forster, F. M., Klove, H., Peterson, W. G., and Bengzon, A. R. A.: Modification of musicogenic epilepsy by extinction technique. *Trans Am Assoc,* 1965.
22. Charany, J. A., Fischbold, H., Messimy, R., and Arfel-Capdevielle: Etude clinique et EEG d'un cas d'epilepsie provoque electivement par le lecture. *Rev Neurol, 95*:381, 1956.

23. Forster, F. M., Hansotia, P., Cleeland, C. S., and Ludwig, A.: A case of voice-induced epilepsy treated by conditioning. *Neurology,* *19*:325, 1969.

24. White, J. C.: A case of reading epilepsy with observations on the effect of sleep and fasting on EEG correlates. *Electroencephalogr Clin Neurophysiol, 28*:510, 1970.

25. Ingvar, D. H. and Nyman, G. E.: Epilepsia arithmetices. A new psychologic trigger mechanism in a case of epilepsy. *Neurology, 12*:282, 1962.

26. Alajouanine, T. et al.: A propas d'un cas d'épilepsie déclenché par la lecture. *Rev Neurol, 101*:463, 1959.

27. Mayersdorf, A. and Marshall, C.: Pattern activation in reading epilepsy. A case report. *Epilepsia, 11*:423, 1970.

CHAPTER 6

EPILEPSY EVOKED BY HIGHER COGNITIVE FUNCTIONS; DECISION-MAKING EPILEPSY

T HE PRECEDING CHAPTER discussed reading or language epilepsy and demonstrated why this type of reflex epilepsy should be considered an involvement of higher nervous system functions, especially in the realm of communication. In this chapter, consideration will be given to seizure evocations which also lie in the realm of higher cognitive functions but which primarily involve decision making. That these two forms of reflex epilepsy are closely related is indicated by the second case in this chapter whose seizures were evoked by reading as well as by decision making.

CASE 1. This twenty-year-old United States Air Force Airman had seizures evoked by decision making. He was studied at Travis Air Force Base and at the Epilepsy Center of the University of Wisconsin. This patient has previously been reported.[1]

The patient had his first seizure at the age of eighteen, preceded by an aura which he described as a shaking feeling. He realized he was beginning to jerk slightly, and an "electric shock shot through" him. Following this, he collapsed on the floor and was told by friends that he "shook all over." He was not incontinent of urine or feces and did not injure himself, but postictally he was confused for several hours.

Since that first seizure, he noted that he had myoclonic jerking whenever he concentrated on some task. When this occurred however, if he immediately sat down and tried to "make my mind go blank," he could prevent the further progress of the seizures. He also noted that the lack of sleep, fatigue, a moderate or greater use of alcohol, and lack of food make him more susceptible to having these minor seizures.

He has had seizures while filling out insurance forms, playing cards (especially playing cards when money and some drinking were involved), during glucose tolerance tests, during military briefing, but most frequently and reliably when he was playing chess.

His past medical history was negative. His birth and delivery were normal, and he had suffered no head trauma. His family history was negative for epilepsy.

General physical and neurological examinations were normal, and the routine laboratory studies were normal.

Neuropsychological evaluation revealed that the patient was functioning in the upper end of the average range of intelligence on the Wechsler Adult Intelligence Scale, and was right handed, right eyed, and right footed, indicative of left cerebral dominance. He had mild difficulty on tests of sustained attention and concentration; a mild asymmetry was noted on tests of motor speed and strength, with the left hand performing slightly more poorly than the right.

RESEARCH STUDIES

When the patient was studied in the research laboratory, seizures were induced by various decision-making techniques, and these were associated with EEG changes.

This patient had two types of dysrhythmia. One of these was a very small low voltage spiking dysrhythmia lasting a fraction of a second (Fig. 30A). This occurred in the routine and sleep records, when he was recorded under sensory restriction conditions, and, indeed, during all situations under which he was recored in the laboratory. This was considered a minor dysrhythmia and was not felt to be not clinically significant, since at no time were there objective or subjective clinical changes associated with this dysrhythmia.

The major dysrhythmia was a large, generalized burst of atypical three per second wave and spike disturbances lasting for several seconds and beginning at either the F3 (Fig. 30B)

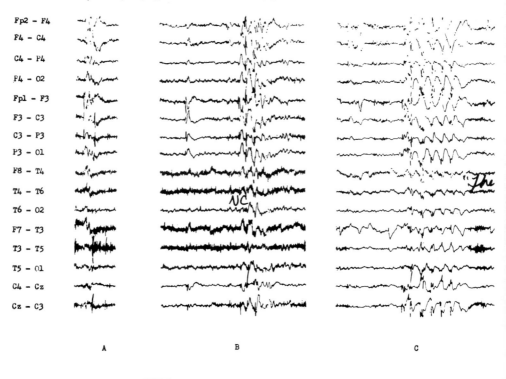

	Fp2 – F4
	F4 – C4
	C4 – P4
	P4 – O2
	Fp1 – F3
	F3 – C3
	C3 – P3
	P3 – O1
	F8 – T4
	T4 – T6
	T6 – O2
	F7 – T3
	T3 – T5
	T5 – O1
	C4 – Cz
	Cz – C3

A   B   C

1 Sec | 50 uV

Figure 30. Seizures evoked by decision making. The EEG dysrhythmias occurring in Case 1. Figure 30A shows minor dysrhythmia which occurred spontaneously in sensory restriction and during decision making. This was never accompanied by objective or subjective clinical manifestations. Figure 30B and Figure 30C show the major dysrhythmia, occurring only during decision making and almost invariably associated with objective and/or subjective clinical manifestations. This dysrhythmia could begin in either the left (Fig. 30B) or right (Fig. 30C) frontal regions. *Arch Neurol, 32*:54, 1975.

or the F4 electrode (Fig. 30C). This type of disturbance was seen only in the evoking conditions and is referred to as "the dysrhythmia."

The patient's seizures were myoclonic in type, affecting arms, head, trunk, and legs, although not necessarily all in a given seizure. Sometimes only the arms or legs were involved. In some of the seizures, the myoclonic phase was subjective rather than objective, i.e. the patient felt the seizure, but the laboratory personnel could not observe movement. There is no doubt they were real, since the subjective seizures coincided with the major EEG dysrhythmia. At no time was a major motor seizure witnessed, although such have been well documented in his history.

The occurrence of seizures during the playing of chess was confirmed repeatedly during these studies (Fig. 31). It was determined that the seizures and dysrhythmia were not visually induced. The patient was tested for visually induced epilepsy with patterns and stroboscopic stimulation, and no dysrhythmia or seizures occurred. Also, when he played chess in the laboratory with one eye covered (monocular testing) or blindfolded, seizures and dysrhythmia occurred (Fig. 32).

The seizure evocation was not the result of tactile stimulation. When the audiovisual tapes were reviewed, it was apparent that

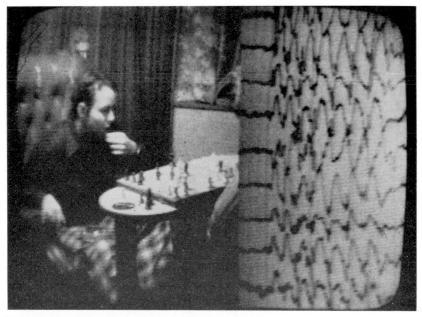

Figure 31. Decision-making epilepsy. Case 1. Atypical spike-wave dysrhythmia evoked by decision making during game of chess. Note concerned attitude of patient. Dysrhythmia accompanied by myoclonic jerking of head and upper extremities.

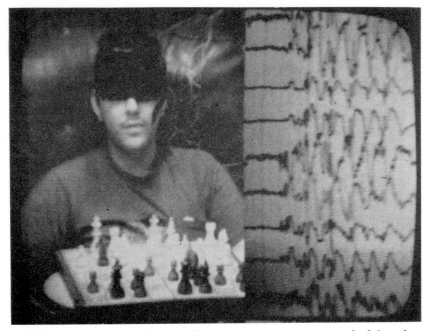

Figure 32.   Decision-making epilepsy.   Case 1.   Seizures evoked by playing chess blindfolded, thus possible role of visual clues is excluded.   Note dysrhythmia begins in left frontal regions (channels 5 and 6 of EEG).

there was no temporal relationship between tactile stimuli and the occurrence of the dysrhythmia and seizures. Most of the seizures occurred when the patient was contemplating a move and when his fingers were not on a chessman. Moreover, in a game played blindfolded, he did not touch the pieces or board, but seizures nevertheless occurred. These observations rule out a tactile stimulus as an evoking factor during the chess game.

In only one of the multiple games of chess that he played during the period of study was there no dysrhythmia. This was when an unusual set (Spanish Renaissance), with which he was unfamiliar, was employed. However, during the second game with this set, seizures occurred. This observation raised the possibility that the seizure incidence might be altered by distraction. This, however, could not be established. While playing chess, he was asked to signal the occurrence of seizures, and he did this without altering the incidence of seizures. Also while playing chess, he was asked to listen to music being played and to identify it. These were very short musical numbers and, even though he was identifying the numbers, seizures occurred. He was also asked to continually whistle a particular song for a period of time. He did this quite well, but the whistling did not prevent the occurrence of the seizures during the chess game. Distraction therefore did not inhibit the occurrence of dysrhthmias or of seizures.

The playing of checkers in the laboratory did not cause seizures. Checkers, of course, was very easy for him. He engaged in a card game with one investigator only. There was no real challenge, no money was at stake, and no alcohol was imbibed; no seizures occurred. By history, it was previously noted that he had had seizures while playing cards for money and when drinking.

When given complex mathematical problems, especially division, seizures occurred. These could be induced either when he was writing the solution to the problem or when he was computing it "in his head," even when blindfolded so that there was no visual input. Simple multiplications, e.g. two digits by one, did not evoke dysrhythmia or seizures.

The neuropsychological testing, except the Halsted category test, was monitored in the Research Laboratory. During the monitored testing, the only times the patient had seizures were with solving mathematical problems and in the Wechsler block subdesign test, at a point when he was faced with ten blocks and was having difficulty putting them in order.

Only two other situations occurred in which he had seizures or dysrhythmia in the laboratory. The first of these was when working on his menu. A seizure occurred during a decision-making task involving two main entrees, neither of which he liked. The second instance in which seizures occurred was when he was asked to write from memory the Pledge of Allegiance to the Flag and the "Star Spangled Banner." When informed by the technician that he had left out a sentence in the National Anthem, he had a burst of dysrhythmia. He was quite concerned about this failure because of his military, patriotic self-concept.

He had no seizures or dysrhythmia while reading, writing

from memory, or copying a nonunderstood language. Reading numbers alone did not evoke a seizure, but when he read the logarithmic tables he had difficulty with the symbols for sign, cosign, degree, and minute. When he tried to employ these signs together with the numbers, he had evoked dysrhythmias; when told simply to read the numbers, this did not occur.

It became evident that the evoking factor in his seizures was primarily decision making. The decision had to be a relatively complex one, not a simple yes/no or on/off decision. The decisions, moreover, had to be sequential and related. For example, during the MMPI testing each decision is apparently independent of the others, and this evoked no problems.

The evoking decisions were usually as in chess, nonverbal, although seizures could occur with verbal symbols also, for example, on the menu. The verbal stimuli could be written as on the menu, or oral as when faced with his error in the National Anthem. It should be noted that menu selection requires some sequential planning between courses, and the sequence in sentences in the National Anthem were the source of the sequential factor in the observation.

Moreover, some tension or anxiety was necessary regarding the result of the decision. This latter point was well exemplified during the course of the chess games. A chess game was charted as played and marked for the incidence of seizures (Fig. 33). No seizures occurred in the opening moves until his opponent captured a piece. Later, when another piece was captured and he was presented with an imminent threat, he "innocently" attempted an illegal move and seven seizures occurred while he delayed for an inordinately long period of time over his next move. Later in the game, when he was on the offense and definitely winning, no seizures occurred. In games that he lost, when he was on the defense and when the situation was so utterly hopeless and that there was no longer any concern about the future of the game, no seizures occurred. Replaying the game in Fig. 31 on command and without decision making evoked no seizures.

To test the role of tension or anxiety alone, he was given a cold pressor test. His right foot was immersed in icewater for

White (Patient)	Black (R.H.)		White (Patient)	Black (R.H.)
1. K P - K$_3$	K P - K$_4$		* Delay	
2. Q - KB$_3$	K Kt. - K B$_3$	18.	Q - K$_7$	Kt x P
3. Q K P - Q K$_3$	Q P - Q$_4$	19.	K R - Q$_2$	*Kt - K$_5$
4. Q B - Q K$_2$	Q K - Q B$_3$	*20.	P - Q B$_4$	B - Q R$_3$
5. Q B x K P	Kt x B*	21.	P - Q R$_4$	K B$_6$ ck (not a real threat)
6. Q Kt - Q B$_3$	Q B - Q K$_5$	22.	K - Q B$_2$	P x P*
7. Q - K B$_4$	K B - Q$_3$	23.	K x Kt	R - Kt$_1$
8. K B - Q K$_5$ (ck)	P - Q B$_3$	24.	Q - K B$_7$	P - Q K$_4$
*9. P - Q$_4$	Q - Q R$_4$	25.	R - Q$_7$	R - Q Kt
*10. K Kt - K$_2$	B x Kt*	26.	R - Q$_1$	P - K R$_3$
** (long delay in game)		27.	Q - K Kt$_6$	P x P
* Tried illegal move with error ****			* Delay	
11. P x Kt	B x B*	28.	P x P	P - Q B$_4$
12. P x B	Q x Kt (ck)	29.	R - Q$_6$	R - Q Kt$_1$
13. K - Q$_1$	O - O	30.	R x B	R - Q K$_6$ ck
14. R - K$_1$	Q - K$_2$ (ck)	31.	K - Q$_2$	R - Q K$_1$
15. R x Q	Kt - K$_5$*	32.	R x P	R x R
* Delay		33.	Q x R$_{mate}$	
16. Q - K$_5$	P - K B$_3$			
17. Q - K$_6$ (ck)	K - R$_1$			

* Indicates occurrence of seizure in patient
and shows whether before or after a move

Figure 33. Plotting of chess game showing occurrence of seizures. Seizures occurred only in response to threatening moves or on errors by patient. When this game was replayed without direct concern but on command and calling for each move, no seizures occurred.

five minutes. This caused a three-degree drop in skin temperature and a rise in systolic blood pressure. It was obviously successful as a stressor test. However, no seizures and no significant EEG dysrhythmia occurred during this test. He was not given any choices or decisions to make.

To test the role of stress and nonsequential decision making, he was pressed, after some preliminary training, to name as rapidly as possible all words he could think of beginning with the letter "z." He did not follow any logical pattern, but gave a random scattering. He was pressured for time and for possible errors throughout this test. No seizures and no dysrhythmia occurred. The latter two observations rule out the role of stress alone and the importance of the sequential decision making.

CASE 2. This patient also appears as Case 9 in the chapter on reading epilepsy. He is a classical example of reading epilepsy but has in addition dysrhythmia and seizures under conditions similar to those of the preceding patient.

The patient was a thirty-one-year-old married accountant. At the age of fourteen years, while playing football, he suffered a head injury. He did not lose consciousness but was amnesic for about three hours. About one month later, he had a seizure which was characterized by loss of consciousness for approximately ten minutes. No postical phenomena were observed, nor were tonic movements. Over the next several years, he had eight of these seizures, and two years after that, until the age of nineteen years, he had occasional flinging of his arms back, with loss of consciousness but not falling to the floor. With none of these were there tonic-clonic movements. He did bite his tongue on several occasions, but he was never incontinent. Postictal fatigue or confusion were never reported.

Upon close questioning, it became evident that most of his major seizures occurred while he was playing cards and concentrating upon a card hand. They were not related to dealing or shuffling and occurred only when he was contemplating a play or in the actual play, and only when he was looking at the cards.

The patient was studied first for the possibility of visually induced epilepsy. The entire range of strobscopic stimulations evoked no seizures either with eyes open or closed. He was presented with the patterns, and no seizure or dysrhythmia was evoked. Also, no dysrhythmia occurred on eye closure or eye opening.

His reading epilepsy was well-documented. When reading nonmemorized reading materail, within eight and one-half minutes he had clinical seizures with a left frontal temporal spiking dysrhythmia. The presence of reading epilepsy was established as indicated in Chapter 5.

The role of card playing was next tested. He was involved

in a game of euchre, a relatively simple card game, with two of the laboratory technicians. They played for twenty-five minutes without any seizures or dysrhythmia being evoked. He then observed that he played cards with his children and in children's games never had any difficulty playing, for they are relatively simple. He was later engaged in a bridge game, replaying hands from the newspaper articles on bridge. Bifrontal spiking discharges were evoked. There was no clinical seizure, however. He observed a game of chess and had no clinical manifestations, and his EEGs at this time were also normal. He then entered into a game of chess, and spiking dysrhythmias were evoked. Following this, he was again exposed to reading material, and the classic reading epilepsy was again demonstrated.

The studies in this second patient were not as detailed as in the first case. The observation time was limited to a single day in the laboratory. Nevertheless, there can be no doubt as to the occurrence of reading epilepsy in this patient and the occurence of dysrhythmias during periods of concentration in complex games. There is also a history of major seizures occurring during such activities, and these facts indicate that this patient has both reading epilepsy and seizures evoked by concentration and decision making.

Symonds,[2] in a review article, mentions that the playing of chess in one of his patients, and the adding of figures in another, were very likely to end in an attack. Ingvar and Nyman[3] report an instance of epilepsy evoked by mathematical computations. Symonds also quotes Bingel's[4] report of a patient who had seizures if he played cards for longer than two hours. Gomez and Escueta[5] comment on a physician patient who had seizures when playing mahjong.

Ch'en, Ch'in and Ch'u, in a more detailed study, report four patients with seizures occurring with chess and card playing.[6] They too rule out the role of visual or tactile stimuli as evoking factors in their patients. They comment on the possible role of proprioceptive impulses from the restless movements and tension, and the emotional factors aroused by a chess game. They note that in one of their four patients, reading, calculation, puzzles, and memory tests did not induce any clinical seizures or electroencephalographic changes. They do not report whether or not they tried these procedures in the other three patients. The authors concluded that the epileptic seizures induced by chess and card games might be considered as the most complex pattern of the reflex epilepsy so far discovered.

This author and his colleagues concur in the opinion of the complexity and feel that the stimulus lies in the higher cognitive functions, under very specific conditions. It is possible that the three factors of (a) complex decision making, (b) sequential decision making, and (c) stress, may vary somewhat in their threshold effect. In other words, if the stress is greater, perhaps the sequential nature need not be as strong and the complexity of the particular decision not as evident. This is suggested in Case 1 by the seizure evoked by the failure to recall one line of the National Anthem in this particularly stressful situation for an Air Force enlistee.

Particularly noticeable also are the various factors in day-to-day life that influence seizure incidence as remarked upon by Case 1. It is not unusual to find a patient who realizes that lack of sleep, the use of alcohol, or the lack of food increases the likelihood of seizures. To have them all come out so clearly in the history of this particular patient raises the question as to whether or not, in these higher forms of reflex epilepsy, these physiological variables may play an even greater role than they do in most instances of epilepsy.

REFERENCES

1. Forster, F. M. et al.: Reflex epilepsy evoked by decision making. *Arch Neurol,* 32:54, 1975.
2. Symonds, C.: Excitation and inhibition in epilepsy. *Brain,* 82:133, 1962.
3. Ingvar, D. H. and Nyman, G. E.: Epilepsia arithmetices. A new psychologic trigger mechanism in a case of epilepsy. *Neurology,* 12:282, 1962.
4. Bingel, A.: Reading epilepsy. *Neurology,* 7:752, 1957.
5. Gomez, G. L. and Escueta, A. V.: Epilepsy in the Phillipines. *J Med* (Phil), 19:318, 1964.
6. Ch'en, Han-Pai, Ch'in, Chen, and Ch'u Chic-Ping. *Chinese Med J,* 84:470, 1965.

CHAPTER 7

EPILEPSY EVOKED BY
SOMATOSENSORY STIMULATION

In THIS CHAPTER are discussed patients whose seizures were evoked by somatosensory stimulation of a part of the body. While cases of this type have been known for a century, they are relatively uncommon. Dunsmore, in 1874,[1] probably gave the earliest description, and his case resembled that later described by Hughlings Jackson,[2] in 1887, of a seven-year-old boy who had a seizure whenever his head was touched, provided there was an element of surprise.

The present study includes four cases of somatosensory-evoked epilepsy. Based upon observations of these cases and of those reported in the literature, the somatosensory-evoked cases can be divided into two groups. The first is characterized by the necessity for an element of startle, and the evoking stimulus must be a sudden, brisk tap administered to a particular part of the body. Such patients have also been reported by Gowers,[3] Spratling,[4] Allen,[5] and Vizoli et al.[6]

In the second group, the stimulus need not be unexpected and consists of a more prolonged type of somatosensory stimulus. Cases of this type have been described by Goldie and Green[7] and Woodcock.[8] In the latter case, the child had seizures upon removal of the right stocking! Penfield and Erickson[9] described a patient whose seizures began with salivation, were induced by pressing on the left gum, and were accompanied by electrical discharges in the lower portion of the right postcentral gyrus. Table X summaries the data gained from the study patients.

TABLE X

SOMATOSENSORY-EVOKED EPILEPSY

Case	Stimulation Characteristic	Location of Stimulation	Startle	Type of Seizure	EEG Dysrhythmia
1	Brisk tap	Left shoulder	+	Absence	Right central s/sw
2	Brisk tap or skin shock	Right thigh	+	Absence	Left temporal spike
3	Repeated rubbing	Left hand	0	Psycho-motor	None defined
4	Rubbing	Face, R>L	0	General-ized clonic	Right frontal s to gen s/w

+ Indicates startle necessary.
* Indicates startle not necessary.

SOMATOSENSORY-EVOKED EPILEPSY: BRISK AND STARTLING STIMULUS

CASE 1. This case has been reported previously.[10] The patient, a girl four years of age, had been studied by the author in the Epilepsy Clinic of the Jefferson Hospital.

At the age of five months, the mother noted that the girl's left arm was not being employed normally. Shortly after this, the first seizure occurred, beginning with twitching of the left corner of the mouth, spreading to involve the external angle of the eye, and then to clonic movements of the left arm and leg. The attack lasted about one minute, was not associated with loss of consciousness, but afterwards the patient was listless and drowsy. These Jacksonian motor seizures occurred ten times and were followed by a postictal paresis of the left arm and leg varying in severity from mild to complete paralysis and lasting from a few minutes to five days. In several seizures the patient complained of pain in the left arm. These Jacksonian seizures were controlled by the use of anticonvulsant medication.

Beginning at the age of seventeen months, the patient's mother noted that tapping of the girl's left shoulder produced a transient attack. These attacks occurred many times a day. Normal play with other children was impossible because of the frequent attacks induced by contact.

The family history was negative for epilepsy. The patient was third in birth order, born at full-term on September 19, 1943 after an uneventful pregnancy and labor. At the age of fifteen months, she had an attack of pain in the right ear, followed by free purulent discharge. At the age of twenty-eight months she had measles. The course of this illness was uneventful.

Physical examination was normal. Neurological examination revealed that the left foot dragged slightly in walking and the left arm was carried in semiflexion. The patient was unable to hop on the left foot. The left thigh, arm, hand, and shoulder were smaller than the right. The deep tendon reflexes were decreased in the left arm and increased in the left leg. There was plantar extension on the left.

RESEARCH STUDIES

Tapping of the left shoulder produced a transient loss of consciousness with forward flexion of the body, resulting in falling if the patient was unsupported (Fig. 34), upward deviation of the eyes and staring, and elevation of the arms, particularly the left. Induced seizures were always momentary. Objects held in the hand were dropped during a seizure. If the patient was aware that she was about to be tapped, an attack was less likely to occur. The optimum site of stimulation was over the posterior aspect of the acromion process on the left, although tapping over the left scapula also frequently produced an attack. Tapping below the costal cage never induced an attack, but occasionally (about once in eight or nine tries), tapping of the right should produced a seizure.

Light touch with a brush or vibration (C128) were ineffective stimuli, but light pinprick occasionally produced an attack. Jostling such as that induced by bumping into her chair produced attacks. Tapping while asleep produced the same elevation of arms and deviation of eyes, although the response was not as uniformly elicited while asleep as when awake.

Repeated electroencephalographic studies between April, 1946 and July, 1947 revealed some four to six per second activity

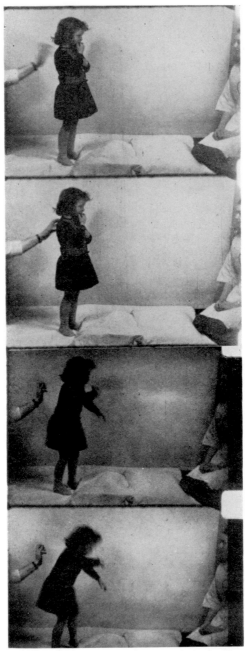

Figure 34.   Somatosensory-evoked epilepsy.   Case 1.   Frames from movie showing akinetic drop attack induced by a brisk, unexpected tap administered to the left shoulder.

from frontocentral regions with eight per second activity in the occipital tracings. Sensory-induced attacks were accompanied by a large evoked potential consisting of a single diphasic spike usually followed by a high voltage slow wave of approximately one third of a second in duration (Fig. 35). This abnormal discharge did not occur if the patient did not have an attack due to awareness of the application of the stimuli, application of inadequate stimuli, or application of the appropriate stimulus to some other region, e.g. the thigh. The initial large evoked potential was occasionally followed by a series of rhythmic waves. From the scalp leads, maximum voltage appeared to be over the right superior central region.

The intensive use of all the anticonvulsant medications available at that time in no way affected the frequency or severity

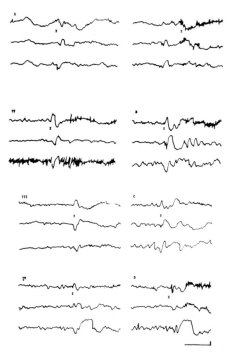

Figure 35. Somatosensory epilepsy. Case 1. EEG changes evoked by tapping left shoulder. 1946 EEG using three channel EEG (Grass). Tracings I to IV are saggital, beginning right lateral. Tracings A to D are coronal, right to left. "X" indicates administration of stimulus.

of the sensory-induced seizures. On February 27, 1948, Doctor Wilder Penfield operated upon the patient at the Montreal Neurological Institute. The right hemisphere appeared normal except that there was, in the central region, a capillary hemangioma or nevus that spread along the fissure of Rolando, appearing much like a dark red strip of carpet. Above, it widened out as it approached the fissure of Sylvius. The hemangioma seemed to be leptomeningeal. There was no evidence of abnormal vascularization of the underlying gyri.

The position of the hemangioma was chiefly postcentral. The postcentral gyrus was quite narrow in its upper extent where it was markedly scarred in the vicinity of the falx. As it passed downward, the gyrus became still narrower and was actually buried in the central fissure. It extended as a submerged microgyrus down to within one and one-half centimeters above the fissure of Sylvius, at which point it seemed to end.

In the upper central region, the hemangioma spread onto the precentral gyrus in a small area, but the underlying motor gyrus was not atrophic. Next to the longitudinal sinus there were adhesions to the dura, suggesting that there had been a small local hemorrhage at some time from the vascular carpet.

Electrocorticography was performed by Doctor Herbert Jasper. Within the hemangiomatous area there was a depression in the voltage of activity. Sharper waves of higher voltage were obtained from a local cortical area about the central fissure. Since no spikes were observed, the sharp waves were considered to have arisen from some nearby focus, possibly deep to the surface. The atrophied postcentral gyrus was later found to be buried beneath this region.

The electrical activity from other exposed cortical regions, including the cingulate gyrus, was considered to show no definite abnormality.

Evoked potentials of high voltage (over 500 microvolts) were obtained from a restricted postcentral area, only in response to tapping the shoulder (Fig. 36). Tapping the left hand and face produced no such responses. With the electrodes arranged in lines on each side of the central fissure, evoked potentials could be obtained only from a small focus just below the upper one of the two hemangiomatous areas in the postcentral region.

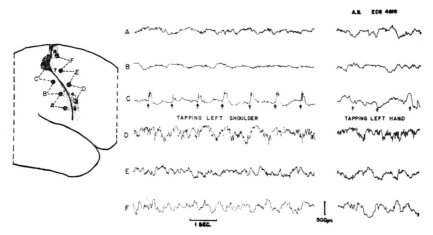

Figure 36. Somatosensory epilepsy. Case 1. Dysrhythmia evoked by stimulation. Electrocorticography by Doctor Herbert H. Jasper. (From *Electroencephalogr Clin Neurophysiol, 1*:349, 1949).

These high-voltage evoked potentials demonstrated a marked facilitation of a local area of the postcentral gyrus. The specificity of this area was clearly indicated by its response only when tapping the shoulder, not when the stimulus was applied to the hand or to the face, although detailed exploration of areas of the body about the shoulder was not carried out.

Doctor Penfield completely removed the postcentral gyrus beginning above at the cingulate fissure. The removal was carried down into the fissure of Sylvius so that the island of Reil was exposed.

The child recovered satisfactorily and was discharged upon recovery from surgery. Somatosensory stimulation failed to elicit any akinetic attacks or EEG abnormalities (Fig. 37). The postoperative left hemiparesis gradually improved over a period of about four weeks.

The patient was continued on phenobarbital for several years, and this was gradually withdrawn. She had no further difficulties until 1971. At the age of twenty-eight, while pregnant and preeclamptic, she had a major motor seizure and was again placed on medication. She has since remained seizure free.

CASE 2. This case has been reported in abstract form.[11] The

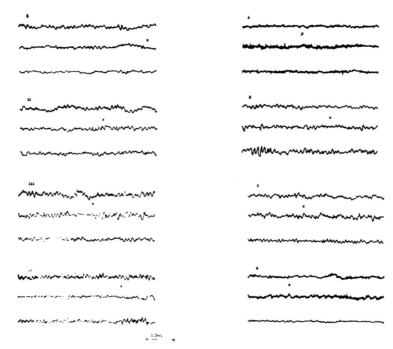

Figure 37. Somatosensory-evoked epilepsy. Case 1. EEG with somato-sensory stimulation after recovery from surgery. Montage as in Figure 35. No evoked dysrhythmia.

patient had a sudden onset of tonic movements of the right extremities, occasionally with incontinence, when an unexpected tactile stimulus was applied to the right thigh or hypogastrium. Seizures of this nature had been present since the age of nineteen years. Her seizure disorder dated from age six years, when generalized cerebral seizures occurred, preceded by a focal component involving the right leg. She had been treated with phenobarbital, hydantoinates, oxyzolidines, and bromide therapy.

In 1959, at age seventeen years, depth electrode recordings performed elsewhere revealed seizure discharges originating independently from the two hemispheres. At that time, pneumoencephalography and left carotid arteriography were reported to be normal. Skin rashes had occurred in association with several anticonvulsant agents including primidone. However, of all anticonvulsant agents, primidone was the most beneficial.

At age nineteen, the patient began to have seizures consisting of stiffening of the right extremities and incontinence, precipitated by an unexpected touch stimulus to the right thigh or over the lower abdominal quadrant.

The family history was negative for neurological disorders. The general physical examination was normal. Neurological examination revealed bilateral horizontal and upward gaze nystagmus, and an equivocal extensor plantar response on the right. The remainder of the neurological examination was within normal limits. Laboratory tests, including chest and skull films and brain scan, were normal.

RESEARCH STUDIES

The research studies can be summarized as follows: the effective stimuli were tactile stimulation or electric skin shocks, which evoked seizures and/or dysrhythmia only when applied to a particular area of the body surface. This included administration of the stimuli to the right thigh, both lateral and medial aspects, and extended up to and included the hypogastrium. Moreover, if the patient was aware of the impending administration of stimulus, the seizure dysrhythmia did not occur. Deliberate self-stimulation did not evoke a dysrhythmia or seizure. The stimuli which failed to evoke seizures included light touch, pinprick, gusts of air, and vibratory stimulation.

The evoked seizures consisted of a generalized myoclonic jerk of the right arm and leg, immediate loss of consciousness, falling to the floor if upright, and often urinary incontinence. The duration of unconsciousness varied from brief episodes lasting only two to three seconds to longer attacks lasting fifteen to twenty seconds. There was definite unconsciousness with loss of pain. This was demonstrated, inadvertently, on one occasion in the laboratory when the patient dropped a lighted cigarette under her thigh during the myoclonic jerk; the laboratory personnel were not aware of it and when she regained consciousness twelve seconds later, it was obvious that she was in pain and she developed a large blister at the point of contact.

The electroencephalographic pattern with these seizures was much less dramatic. There was a sharp spike with a slow wave

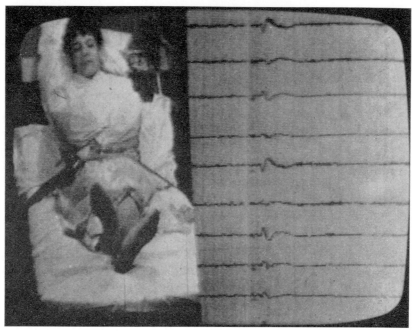

Figure 38.   Somatosensory epilepsy. Case 2. Akinetic seizure evoked by tap administered to right thigh. EEG shows spike and slow wave from left parietal area.

following and occurring especially in the left parietal area (Fig. 38). This was followed by a period of decreased electrical activity (suppression) which persisted throughout the clinical seizure. This decrease in activity was not the result of her opening her eyes in the course of the seizure, for the recording was the same when seizures were evoked in the darkened laboratory.

The presentation of repeated stimuluations to the appropriate body part gave interesting results with significance for treatment techniques. If the repeated stimulations were begun outside the reflexogenous zone, for example, below the knee, and carried into the reflexogenous zone, no seizure or dysrhythmia was elicited. If the repeated stimulations were begun within the zone, but very gently and below threshold, and gradually increased, the previous threshold could be surpassed without seizure or dysrhythmia evocation.

If stimulations at or above threshold were administered re-

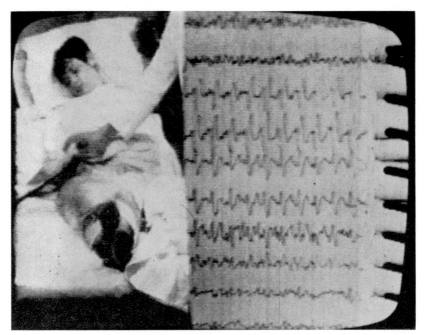

Figure 39. Somatosensory epilepsy. Case 2. Repeated stimulations (approximately three per second) with "driving" of epileptogenic cortex.

peatedly within the reflexogenous zone, the affected cerebral cortex could be driven with a series of spiking discharges (Fig. 39). This was well exemplified at a frequency of three per second. If, however, the rapidity of stimulation was increased to approximately ten per second, no driving occurred (Fig. 40).

These two patients therefore are quite similar in the following aspects: the evoking stimulus had to be unexpected, delivered to a particular part of the body and had to be a brisk tap. In the second case, the evoking stimulus could also be an electric skin shock. In both patients, the clinical seizures were of the akinetic absence type, and the EEG changes consisted primarily of focal slow wave and spike.

SOMATOSENSORY-EVOKED EPILEPSY: WITHOUT STARTLE AND WITH PROLONGED STIMULATION

The following two cases are examples of this form of sensory-evoked epilepsy. In these patients, the stimulus was more com-

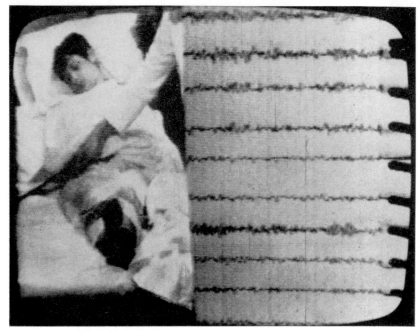

Figure 40.   Somatosensory epilepsy.   Case 2.   Repeated stimulations at faster rate (ten per second) fail to drive cortex.

plex and had to be carried out for a longer period of time than the simple tap in the preceding two patients. Also, the element of startle was not necessary for evocation of the seizure, and the seizures could be definitely self-induced as well.

CASE 3.   This thirty-seven-year-old design engineer had a twenty-seven-year history of focal seizure activity.

The patient had his first seizure at age ten, when he described a shaking of his entire body followed by a period of unconsciousness, then a postictal state of fatigue, but without incontinence or tongue biting. These occurred approximately every one to two weeks, and the patient was hospitalized in Caro State Hospital, Michigan, where he was begun on diphenylhydantoin 300 mg per day and phenobarbital 15 mg three times a day.

Commencing at the age of thirteen, the patient had episodes of "tightening in the hands," shaking of his left arm and hand, all of which occurred nocturnally. These increased in frequency through the next five years, and at the age of eighteen, the patient noted an aura of heightened sensitivity in the left palm, occurring thirty to sixty minutes prior to the flexing of his fingers, shaking of hand and arm, and tonic extension of his arm at the elbow. This activity always occurred when he was resting. After age twenty-five, the frequency of these episodes increased to two per week, and about this time the patient noted he was able to stimulate this focal, left-sided seizure activity by stroking the area of the left palm during the period of heightened sensitivity in this area. Since the age of twenty-five, the patient's seizure incidence varied considerably. He could have months in which he was seizure free, or he might have as many as several seizures per day. He did, however, have some seizure activity almost nightly while asleep. These were described by his wife as extension of the left arm, occasionally accompanied by leg movement. During this time he had been self-stimulating his left palm to induce a seizure in the morning so that he would be able to go to work without fear of a seizure. He had learned that he has a postictal refractory period which made it very unlikely that he would have a subsequent seizure during the day.

Past medical history revealed that he had the usual childhood diseases. At the age of six, however, he was "completely para-lyzed" and was bedridden for six months at home. He was unable to feed himself and could move only his head. It was not possible to obtain medical records for this period. This may have been an attack of rheumatic fever, as suggested by the subsequent removal of his tonsils and adenoids and a prolonged period of penicillin therapy.

The general physical examination was normal. On neuro-logical examination, there was decreased swinging of the left arm on walking, and the patient held his head to the right. On finger-to-finger-to-nose test there was slight dyssynergia on the left. Hand grip was decreased on the left, and finger tapping was slower on the left. The patient's left heel of his shoe was worn more than the right, although his gait appeared normal. The remainder of the neurological examination was normal.

The laboratory and X-ray studies and brain scan were normal. The EEGs in the resting, awake, and in the sleep state were normal. Neuropsychological testing of the patient failed to reveal any evidence of substantial impairment of abilities dependent upon the organic integrity of the cerebral hemispheres. A motor pattern supported by mild sensory findings suggested an area of mild but consistent impairment of cortical functioning in the posterior right frontal area. The pattern on the motor tests suggested that this impairment was related to the primary motor area of the right hemisphere. The patient's MMPI profile was normal.

RESEARCH STUDIES

The patient was studied daily in the research laboratory. During the patient's study, no seizure activity was noted to occur except during periods of special testing. In the beginning, various types of stimulation were employed in attempts to induce a seizure. Electric shock to the skin of the left palmar surface failed to evoke a seizure or dysrhythmia. Manipulating the left hand with the right or rubbing it with a hard metallic object, such as a coin or cigarette lighter, failed to evoke a seizure. A wood rasp was used and found to be effective in producing seizures.

When the AV tape recordings of these seizures were reviewed and compared, the seizures were found to be quite stereotyped. In these seizures he would say "I've got it," meaning that he knew that he was going to have a seizure and would then grasp his left arm with his right, slump down in the chair, turn his head to the side (usually right), and make mouthing movements; his eyes were open and staring, and there was no response to verbal commands. This would last about one minute. Clinically these looked very much like partial complex or psychomotor seizures. He, however, while unable to respond to commands, did recall numbers given to him or names of animals or similar verbal stimuli, but not always accurately. He might occasionally miss a number or miss a name, but for the most part there was no great disturbance of consciousness. Postictally he was entirely clear and would pick up the interrupted count as soon as the seizure was over. Postically he had an increment in his usual mild weakness of the left arm. This was documented on AV tape by a drift in the left arm in space, decrease of digital movements in the left upper extremity, and slight hyperreflexia.

No specific or definitive EEG changes were noted with the seizure or prior to it. During the actual seizure there was a great deal of muscle artifact. Nasopharyngeal leads were put in place and a seizure induced, but no abnormality was noted in the recordings from the nasopharyngeal electrodes.

Since he had nocturnal seizures, a prolonged sleep recording was done. During this, on two occasions, he suddenly sat up, grasped his left knee with his left arm (unaware of what exactly transpired), but again, no EEG changes occurred. There was no manipulation of the left hand prior to or during the seizure. On one occasion while asleep, he rubbed the dorsum of his hand for several strokes, but no seizure occurred. (The seizures only occurred from palmar stimulation.)

The absence of EEG changes could raise the question of pseudoseizures. However, the classical appearance of the seizures as viewed on the AV tape recording, the postical weakness, the postical refractory period and the lack of secondary gain (the seizures he daily induced at home during the morning were to prevent seizures during the day), and seizures during sleep all support the contention that these were true seizures. The EEG focus was not available by recording from scalp or nasopharyngeal electrodes. Deep electrodes were not implanted since there was no indication for surgical ablation.

Hypnosis was attempted, since there are previous reports (including Case 10, Chapter 3) of the induction of reflex epilepsy in the hypnotic state. Under hypnosis, when told that he was rubbing the rasp, the patient manipulated his hand in space as though the rasp were in its usual position, but no seizure could be elicited. Hypnosis did not seem to have any potential for therapy. He was told that, upon being aroused, he would not have a seizure the first time that he was stimulated, but he did have a seizure on the first stimulation, thus indicating that hypnosis would not be effective as a means of blocking the occurrence of the seizures.

Case 4. This patient is another example of specific, non-startling somatosensory-evoked epilepsy. This fifteen-year-old, female high school student had seizures since the age of thirteen.

At that time and during the week of her first menstrual period, she had three episodes, each in the morning before breakfast, consisting of lightning-like jerking of her arms and hands. These lasted from one to two minutes. During these spells the patient would stare and not communicate, and objects fell from her hands. Postictally she was upset and cried but was oriented and not tired. The seizures continued at the rate of about three per week. Nine months later she had her first major motor seizure which occurred while she was talking on the telephone.

Since that time she had averaged three major motor seizures per month, without aura. The movements were clonic and symmetrical in all four extremities with abnormal posturing in her arms. She became cyanotic and had bitten her tongue, and also had been incontinent of urine. Postictally she was slightly disoriented, weak, very tired, and had throbbing headaches.

Many of her seizures occurred while the patient had her hand or hands in contact with her face, for example while telephoning or combing her hair. Her mother noted on three occasions that she had major motor seizures while brushing her teeth. On one occasion when she was having a minor motor attack, her mother put a moist, warm washcloth on her face, and immediately the youngster had a major seizure.

There was a family history of seizures; two first cousins, one paternal and one maternal. One of these had cerebral palsy and polio. There was no other family history of neurological disease.

The patient was the seventh of eight children. Pregnancy, delivery, and development were within normal limits. There was no history of head injury or central nervous system infection. The past history was negative.

The general physical examination was entirely within normal limits, and the neurological examination was also negative, except her calculations were thought to be poor. Her judgment, recent and remove memory, and instant recall were within normal limits. Her affect was immature and proverb interpretation was concrete. Examination of her gait was normal, including walking on heels, toes, tandem, and hopping.

The laboratory tests were normal, including skull X rays, brain scan, and results from neuropsychological examination.

RESEARCH STUDIES

In this patient, the research studies were directed primarily toward the possibility of somatosensory evoking factors.

During the course of applying the electrodes for the first EEG, the patient had what was thought to be a spontaneous seizure. During the recordings a half hour or so later, the author washed her face with warm water and dried it, and had her brush her teeth and comb her hair as well as she could with electrodes in place. No seizure and no dysrhythmia occurred. On each of the next two days while electrodes were being applied, "spontaneous" seizures occurred. It was apparent that these were probably not spontaneous but somatosensory-evoked for they occurred when the first few electrodes were put in place, fastened with collodion, and compressed air directed to the collodion. The frontal electrodes were the first applied. This raised the possibility that the ablutions in the laboratory failed to evoke a seizure since she was in the postictal refractory state.

Accordingly, on the fourth morning, the patient was brought to the laboratory and AV taping begun. The posterior electrodes were put in place first, and, as each electrode became functional, the EEG record was obtained from it until all eighteen electrodes were put in place. No difficulty occurred until the seventeenth electrode was being placed in position and filled with saline over the right frontal area (Fig. 41). She had a seizure which was a minor seizure but not a typical petit mal. The EEG dysrhythmia began with spiking discharge at P4. (The F4 electrode was not yet in operation.) The dysrhythmia rapidly progressed into a somewhat atypical three per second wave and spike followed by a series of fast spikes. The seizure was characterized by myoclonic jerking and then tonic extension of the arms with some jerking and clenching at the electrodes with automatism (Fig. 42). It did not progress to a major motor seizure.

During the recording, two spontaneous absence seizures without automatisms occurred (Fig. 43). These were shorter in duration than the other seizures, lasting about six seconds, and

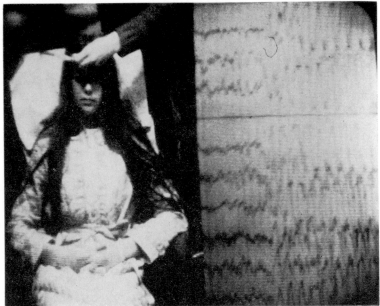

Figure 41. Somatosensory-evoked epilepsy. Case 4. Seizure evoked by electrode placement. Note technician's hand applying the right frontal electrode. The EEG dysrhythmia began at electrode P4, common to the second and third channels.

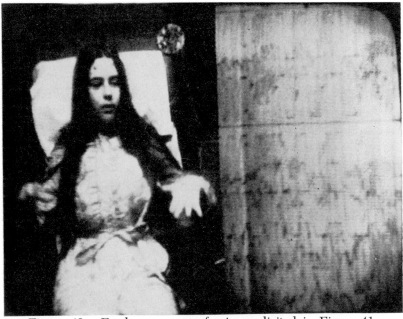

Figure 42. Further progress of seizure elicited in Figure 41.

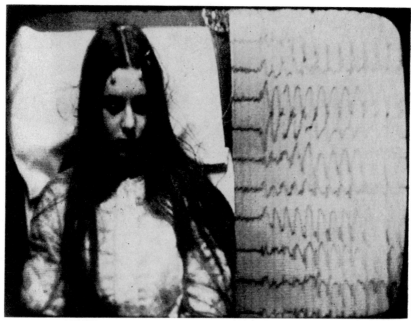

Figure 43. Same patient as in Figures 45 and 46. Spontaneous, non-evoked seizure, typical petit mal in type. Note the dysrhythmia is three per second, and there is no focal onset.

were accompanied by a generalized wave and spike dysrhythmia, with neither the faster activity nor the focal onset.

In summary, this young lady had spontaneous somatosensory-evoked seizures. The occurrence of seizures on four successive days at the time of the application of the frontal electrodes seems beyond the possibility of chance.

The four patients described above represent examples of somatosensory-evoked epilepsy. While seizures evoked by stimulation of this type are uncommon, even rarer forms have been reported.

During the past ten years, seizures occurring upon immersion in water have been described.[12-15] Undoubtedly these are somatosensory-evoked, and the stimulus, as in Cases 3 and 4, is not startling and is not an abrupt stimulus.

Seizures occurring in a woman upon achieving sexual orgasm has been reported by Hoenig and Hamilton.[16] Multiple possible factors are involved here, including the affective. But certainly somatosensory components must play a part.

To date in the laboratory, an opportunity to study the forms of somatosensory epilepsy just described, i.e. immersion and orgasm-induced, has not arisen.

The relationship of the cortical EEG focus to the area of stimulation is in most instances quite clear. This is definitely shown in Case 1 and in numerous of the reported cases in literature. Other evidence is provided by the effect of application of local anesthetics.[18] This, when applied to the appropriate somatic area, may reduce or abolish the attacks, especially when they are produced by a sudden stimulus. Straus[18] demonstrated this by cocainizing the cornea of a patient in whom seizures could be induced by eliciting the right corneal reflex.

Of special interest is the possible relationship of peripheral injury and of cortical lesions to somatosensory-evoked epilepsy. The patient reported by Rae[19] had a penetrating wound of the right frontal lobe and two years later injured his left foot. Following the second injury, stimulation of the left foot evoked seizures. Rae concluded that a peripheral stimulus may excite epilepsy if the corresponding part of the cerebral cortex is in an unstable state. Further evidence is derived from the studies of Vizioli[20] who reports adversive seizures in his patient evoked by rubbing the left side of his neck.

The patients described in the next chapter had their seizures associated with eating. While this may well represent another form of somatosensory-evoked epilepsy as considered by Scollo-Lavizari and Hess,[21] that fact is not clear at the present time, especially in view of the studies carried out on the second patient in the Research Laboratory. Since factors other than somato-sensory may be the evoking factors, the problem of seizures associated with eating is dealt with in a separate chapter.

REFERENCES

1. Dunsmore, J.: *Neurological Fragments.* London, Oxford M. (Oxford U Pr), 1925, p. 114.
2. Jackson, J. H.: *Selected Writings.* Taylor, J. (Ed.). N.Y., Basic, 1958, p. 363.

3. Gowers, E.: *Epilepsy and Other Chronic Convulsive Diseases.* N.Y., Wm Wood, 1885.
4. Spratling, W.: *Epilepsy.* Phila., Saunders, 1904, p. 165.
5. Allen, J.: Observations in cases of reflex epilepsy. *N Z Med J, 44*:135, 1945.
6. Galderon-Gonzalez, R., Hopkins, I., and McLean, W. T.: Tap seizures. *JAMA, 198*:521, 1966.
7. Goldie, L. and Green, J. A.: A study of the psychological factors in a case of sensory reflex epilepsy. *Brain, 82*:505, 1959.
8. Woodcock, C.: A case with complete cessation of fits resembling epilepsy. *Lancet, 2*:60, 1919.
9. Penfield, W. and Erickson, T. C.: *Epilepsy and Cerebral Localization.* Springfield, Thomas, 1941.
10. Forster, F. M., Penfield, W., Jasper, H., and Madow, L.: Focal epilepsy, sensory precipitation and evoked potentials. *Electroencephalogr Clin Neurophysiol, 1*:349, 1949.
11. Forster, F. M. and Cleeland, C. S.: Somato-sensory epilepsy. *Trans Am Neurol Assoc, 94*:268, 1969.
12. Mofenson, H. C., Weymuller, C. A., and Greensher, J.: Epilepsy due to water immersion. *JAMA, 191*:600, 1965.
13. Keipert, J. A.: Epilepsy precipitated by bathing. *Aust Paediatr J, 5*:2444, 1969.
14. Mani, K. S., Copalakrishnan, P. N., and Vyas, J. N.: "Hot water epilepsy"—a peculiar type of reflex epilepsy. A preliminary report. *Neurol India, 16*:107, 1969.
15. Stensman, R. and Ursing, B.: Epilepsy precipitated by hot water immersion. *Neurology, 21*:559, 1971.
16. Hoenig, J. and Hamilton, C. M.: Epilepsy and sexual organs. *Acta Psychiatr Scand, 35*:448, 1960.
17. Lishman, W., Symonds, C., Whitty, W., and Willison, R.: Seizures induced by movement. *Brain, 85*:93, 1962.
18. Strauss, H.: Jacksonian seizures of reflex origin. *Arch Neurol Psychiat, 44*:140, 1932.
19. Rae, J. W.: Case report. Reflex epilepsy and peripheral injury. *J Neurol Neurosurg Psychiatry, 15*:134, 1952.
20. Vizioli, R.: The problem of human reflex epilepsy. In Servit, Z. (Ed.): *Reflex Mechanisms in the Genesis of Epilepsy.* Amsterdam, Elsevier, 1963, p. 85.
21. Scollo-Lavizari, G. and Hess, R.: Sensory precipitation of epileptic seizures. *Epilepsia, 8*:157, 1967.

CHAPTER 8

EPILEPSY RELATED TO EATING

L oss of consciousness associated with deglutition was first described by Soma Weiss.[1] He demonstrated in his patient a vasovagal reflex elicited by food lodged in an esophageal diverticulum. Subsequent reports of other authors[2, 3] add additional cases of syncope associated with swallowing, sometimes with a particular type of food intake, especially carbonated beverages.[4, 5]

Scollo-Lavizzari and Hess[6] described a youngster with episodes of grimacing movements of his mouth and tongue elicited by mastication and swallowing but without disturbance of consciousness.

The author has had the opportunity to study two patients with epilepsy associated with eating. One of these, Case 1 was quite uncooperative, so the studies are limited, but in Case 2 detailed observations were possible, and this patient was the basis of a report presented to the American Neurological Association.[7] In the discussion of that presentation, Stevens[8] reported on a patient with myoclonic jerks associated with swallowing. The following are the resumes of the study patients.

CASE 1. The patient was a seventeen-year-old female with a history of seizures occurring three or four times per day and generally occurring while eating. The seizures consisted of suddenly staring, becoming limp, slumping in her chair or, if standing, falling to the ground. Food was retained in her mouth, and she drooled and was unable to swallow. The seizures lasted approximately thirty seconds. There was unconsciousness, but no tonic-clonic movements, bizarre behavior, or incontinence were associated with the episodes.

The past medical history revealed a diagnosis of arthrogryposis multiplex congenita with multiple operations for the correction

156

of bilateral club feet, displaced patella, and a right dislocated hip. The family history was negative for seizures.

The general physical examination revealed the evidence of her orthopedic problems and surgical corrections, but otherwise was negative. On neurological examination she was alert and oriented. There was weakness of the lower extremities, atrophy of the hand muscles diffusely and bilaterally, and marked atrophy of the calves. She had a waddling gait typical of the Trendelenburg-type gait. The rest of the neurological examination was negative.

The patient was studied in the Research Laboratory where she had, while eating dry cereal, a seizure with abrupt cessation of activity. Her food drooled from her mouth; she was not unconscious but unable to swallow and did not speak. Definite and significant EEG changes occurred with this seizure. Prior to the seizure there was marked muscle artifact. This ceased in the seizure, and there was an abrupt onset of sharp, high amplitude alphalike rhythms with a frequency of eleven per second beginning in the right anterior temporal region. After one second, this became generalized high voltage and sharp, and was followed by postictal slowing. The entire episode lasted two and one-half minutes.

Unfortunately it was not possible to work extensively with this patient because she refused to eat the food which she herself had chosen when placed before her in the laboratory. She removed the electrodes and refused to stay in the laboratory. The aforementioned was the only meal which we were able to serve her. In view of the history of seizures while eating and the demonstration in the laboratory, it is most likely that this patient could have epilepsy associated with eating despite the paucity of our formal laboratory data.

Case 2. This patient was a twenty-one-year-old female who had experienced minor seizures since the age of ten. Most of her seizures were associated with eating, and she rarely ate a meal without having a seizure.

At the age of ten years, the patient began having attacks which consisted of episodes of inability to speak and some involvement of tongue movements without disturbance of consciousness. These attacks lasted from five to ten seconds and occurred about once or twice a day. At age twelve, with some of these episodes, the patient had deviation of the head to the right and some movements of the face and, occasionally, of the right upper extremity. At the age of fifteen, it was noted that her attacks occurred most frequently while eating. The attacks could either be focal, right sided seizures or attacks consisting of aphasia, staring, and drooling with no loss of consciousness. When upright, she had fallen in these episodes. The patient had had only one major motor seizure; this occurred at the age of eleven.

She had been treated with sodium diphenylhydantoin 300 mg per day and primidone 750 mg per day without affecting the frequency of the seizures. Phenobarbital therapy had also been used unsuccessfully in the past.

There was a vague history of seizures in the family of the patient's father, but these could not be more specifically defined. The patient was second in birth order. Prenatal, birth, and developmental histories were normal except that the patient was the product of a difficult delivery and had had an occipital hematoma at the time of birth. She had an unremarkable development, without febrile convulsions. At the age of two, the patient fell down a flight of stairs hitting her head, but there was no definite evidence of loss of consciousness or undue concern at that time on the part of the family.

The general physical examination was normal. The neurological examination was also normal. Routine laboratory studies were normal. Barium esophogram with cinerecording was performed; the esophagus was found to be normal and no diverticulum was found. The testing was done twice. The first study evoked a seizure without change in the esophageal motility.

The patient was seen by Doctor Maxine Bennett of the Ear, Nose, and Throat Department who could find no pharyngeal lesion and who could not evoke a seizure by mechanical stimulation of the nasopharynx.

RESEARCH STUDIES

The patient was studied for three weeks, during which time her breakfast and lunch were served in the laboratory with the customary AV tape recording. Every meal served to her for the first seventeen days induced a seizure. Forty seizures in all were recorded.

The seizures were stereotyped. She suddenly stopped eating (Figs. 44, 45), and occasionally there was some automatic activity. In the first two or three seconds of the seizure she might vigorously stir her cereal, or put her spoon in the orange juice. In all seizures, her head would drop down and her arms, particularly the left, would be raised. Facial movements were markedly decreased, and occasionally her legs moved into extension. She drooled and stopped swallowing. She could recall almost all of the numbers or words presented verbally to her, but occasionally, in a more severe attack, she did have some periods of unconsciousness and could not recall the first few words or numbers presented. She was able to obey quite complex commands such as wiggling the thumb on her left hand (Fig. 46), but was unable to obey the command to "put out your tongue" when interspersed between the other com-

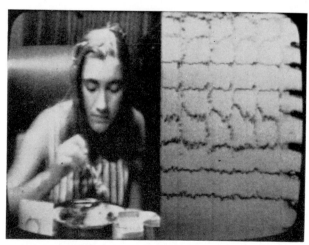

Figure 44. Eating epilepsy. Case 2. Just prior to seizure. Patient is eating. Note facial expression. EEG shows muscle artifact from mastication.

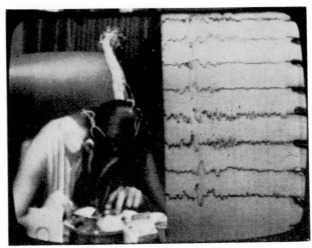

Figure 45. Same patient. Onset of seizure with head dropping. EEG shows last muscle artifact of eating and then a suppression of electrical activity.

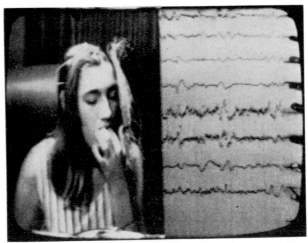

Figure 46. Same patient, one minute after onset of seizure. Trying manually to extrude tongue in response to command "Put out your tongue." Spikes seen in fifth and sixth channels of EEG are from left rolandic area.

mands. In response to the command in reference to her tongue, she sometimes put her fingers into her mouth to open it, pulled her lips apart, and tried to extrude her tongue manually (Fig. 46). Yet immediately before and after this performance, she was able to obey other commands such as "close your eyes, hold and place it in her mouth, chew, and swallow, but no seizure occurred.

From the observations of the seizures and these studies recorded in the laboratory, it was evident that neither the temperature nor the texture of the food played any role in the up your left hand," etc. (Fig. 47). There was therefore either paralysis or apraxia involving the bulbar innervated muscles· during the seizure. The attacks were as short as thirty to forty seconds and as long as six minutes. She rarely had more than one attack in the course of a meal.

The EEG in the early phase of a seizure was somewhat difficult to interpret because of the immediately preceding artifact. The repeated chewing and swallowing caused much muscle artifact. At the onset of the seizure, with the apraxia or paralysis and therefore the loss of muscle artifact, the record appeared to be of lower voltage, and a period of suppression was observed, followed by large spiking dysrhythmia in the left temporal and rolandic regions.

Prolonged voluntary coughing and voluntary swallowing failed to evoke a seizure. The patient was asked to imitate eating and did this for ten minutes, pretending to cut her food

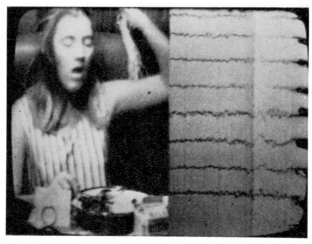

Figure 47. Ten seconds later in same seizure. Patient can lift head and raise left arm on command, but cannot protrude tongue, talk, or swallow. Note expressionless face. EEG still shows some suppression.

induction of seizures. Seizures were induced by hot broth, cold milk, lukewarm cream of wheat and mashed potatoes, dry toast, and hot beefsteak.

To rule out sensory input other than texture and temperature, an anesthetic pressure spray was used to anesthetize her throat. During the process of anesthetizing her throat, on three occasions out of four, seizures resulted. However, dry compressed air spray and a vaporized water spray applied in the same manner did not induce seizures. The chemical used in the spray was not the offender, for when placed on her tongue and allowed to disperse gradually through her nasopharynx, it did not evoke a seizure.

Following the anesthetization of the patient's throat, eating a meal evoked a seizure. This occurred despite the fact that the patient, upon careful testing after the seizure, was unable to identify the various tastes, and her olfactory input was also impaired by the anesthetic spray. A sour lemon drop was thought possibly to be "cherry," and neither the sour aspect nor absence of sweetness were appreciated.

The AV tapes of all her seizures were reviewed to determine if there was a relationship to the phase of deglutition. Some seizures occurred at the very moment of swallowing, others while chewing and before a swallow (one occurred after swallowing), and while talking and reaching for a glass of milk. No relationship therefore could be established to the phase of deglutition.

In the first ten days, no seizures occurred until she had been eating for at least two minutes. However, after this period of time a seizure was observed on the second swallow of broth at the beginning of a meal. There was therefore no apparent relationship to the amount of food intake or to the duration of eating. Since the patient was known to have some seizures while not eating, at least while not eating meals, she was observed and recorded for a period of several hours while reading, listening to music, and typing under some psychological pressure. No seizure occurred in the laboratory under these conditions. It was anticipated that if a seizure had occurred, its relationship to spontaneous swallowing could be determined upon reviewing the AV tapes.

These two patients present examples of seizures evoked by eating. These patients differed considerably from those reported in the literature. The two study patients have paralytic or apractic components to their seizures, involving the cranial or bulbar somatomotor innervation.

While the first patient was not thoroughly studied because of her poor cooperation, the detailed studies on the second patient demonstrate the elusiveness of the evoking factor. Despite careful studies, the nature of the evoking factor could be specified only as eating in its broadest concepts, since texture, temperature, phase of deglutition, time of eating, and taste were all methodically eliminated as specific or aggregate evoking factors.

The second patient and her mother both reported that the patient on occasion had seizures in anticipation of eating. She had been noted to have seizures while opening the refrigerator to remove food for a snack. This was impossible to reproduce in the laboratory. However, this is historical evidence for an anticipatory seizure evocation.

REFERENCES

1. Weiss, S. and Ferris, E. B., Jr.: Adams-Stokes syndrome with transient complete heart block of vagovagal reflex origin mechanism and treatment. *Arch Int Med, 54:*931, 1934.
2. Iolaver, S. and Schwartz, B.: Heart block periodically induced by the swallowing of food in a patient with cardiospasm (vagovagal syncope). *Ann Otol Rhinol Laryngol, 45:*875, 1936.
3. Kopald, H. H., Roth, H. P., Flesher, B., and Pritchard, W. H.: Vago-vagal syncope: report of a case associated with diffuse esophageal spasm. *N Eng J Med, 271:*1238, 1964.
4. Seidel, H. M.: Gaseous soft drinks and symptoms. *Clin Pediatr, 4:*42, 1965.
5. Liske, E.: Personal communications from the School of Areospace Medicine, USAF, Brooke AFB.
6. Scollo-Lavizzari, G. and Hess, R.: Sensory precipitation of epileptic seizures. *Epilepsia, 8:*157, 1967.
7. Forster, F. M.: Epilepsy associated with eating. *Trans Am Neurol Assoc, 96:*106-107, 1971.
8. Stevens, H. S.: In discussion of above. Ref. p. 107.

CHAPTER 9

EPILEPSY EVOKED BY MOVEMENT

SEIZURES ASSOCIATED WITH or evoked by movement were first described by Gowers.[1] Lishman et al.,[2] in 1962, published a very careful review of the cases published up to that time and added an additional seven patients. Since then there have been a number of case reports.[3-12]

The types of seizures evoked by movement have consisted of possible paroxysmal choreo-athetosis (about which there has been some question) and more definitive seizure manifestations of either tonic seizures, with or without loss of consciousness, or clonic-focal seizures.

The choreothetotic induced episodes were questioned as to whether or not they constitute a seizure disorder. But Lishman[2] demonstrated a definite EEG abnormality in one case of the choreo-athetotic induced movement and in two cases with both tonic and athetoid components. Moreover, all three patients responded to anticonvulsant therapy. Therefore, at least some of the cases of induced choreo-athetosis are truly seizure manifestations. It is of note that this form of reflex epilepsy, namely the choreo-athetotic induced by movement, can occur in diseases such as multiple sclerosis.[3, 4]

In movement-induced epilepsy, the evoking factor or factors could be: (a) the motor movement itself, (b) the proprioceptive feedback secondary to the movement, or (c) the very concept of (anticipatory-ideational) motion of the body part.

Doctor Cornelius Van Nuis, of Grand Rapids, Michigan, and the author have had an opportunity to study one patient whose seizures were evoked by movement. The following is a description of this patient.

CASE 1. The patient, an eleven-year-old female, at the age of nine had her first seizure which consisted of a clonic seizure of the right hand. Several months later, a similar seizure occurred with a progression involving the right forearm, and eventually spreading to include the angle of the mouth on the right. These clonic seizures continued to occur two to three times per week and lasted approximately one or two minutes. When they reached their full expression, they were followed by a two hour period of lethargy and occasionally were accompanied by incontinence but not by unconsciousness.

Concurrent with the onset of the seizure disorder, the patient noticed decreased coordination and weakness of the right hand. She became aware that movement of the right upper extremity initiated her seizures.

The past history was noncontributory She was a full term, normal infant. Birth and delivery were uncomplicated and development of all milestones were normal. She started school at the age of four and was an "A" and "B" student. Physical examination was normal except for obesity and a scar on the patient's right arm, the result of a burn suffered during a seizure.

Neurological examination revealed decreased digital facility in the right hand with weakness of extension, abduction, and flexion of the fingers. There was weakness of flexion and extension at the right wrist, but proximal motor power was normal. There was atrophy of the small muscles of the right hand. There were no reflex changes. The lower extremities were completely normal. There was no sensory deficit in the upper or lower extremities with special attention to pinprick, light touch, vibration, position, graphesthesia, stereognosis, and two-point discrimination.

Laboratory studies were normal except for her EEG, which in the resting state was mildly abnormal with generalized disturbances of cerebral function most marked posteriorly and bilaterally. Occasional bursts of delta activity were seen in these regions. Detailed studies, including brain scan, X rays of the skull, pneumoencephalography, and angiography, were all noncontributory.

RESEARCH STUDIES

Specific studies included monitoring while carrying out tests such as writing, and parts of the neuropsychological battery of tests including finger tapping, TPT test, sandpaper discrimination, and other uses of the right and left hand. These activities invariably evoked seizures after thirty seconds to three minutes of activity (Fig. 48). The seizures began with fine clonic movements of the fingers and the thumb, extended to the wrist (Fig. 49) and occasionally to the elbow. At no time did the seizures evoked in the laboratory extend beyond clonic movement at the elbow.

The seizures were accompanied by spiking dysrhythmia in the left motor areas, best seen by an eccentric electrode placed between Cz and C3.

Seizures invariably occurred with the use of the right hand, although on one occasion a seizure occurred when carrying out a neuropsychological test with the left hand. The patient had mirror movements between right hand and left hand. On review-

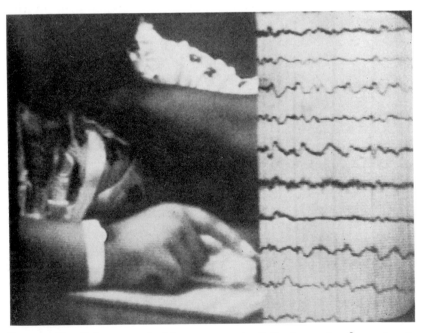

Figure 48. Seizures evoked by movement. Patient pressing finger tapping key during neuropsychologic testing. Clonic movements of right index finger beginning. EEG dysrhythmia in the third channel was obtained from an electrode between C3 and CZ electrodes.

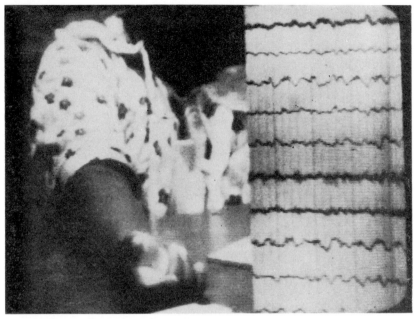

Figure 49. Same patient. Hand in supine position clonic movements of fingers and wrist. EEG dysrhythmia as above.

ing the AV tape, at that particular time, her right hand had sunk deeply into her lap so that her fingers could not be seen, and it was not known whether the right fingers were moving in accord with activities of the left hand. She was given tasks with prolonged activity involving the left hand and with the accompanying associated movements of the right fingers. These associated movements failed to evoke seizures.

The possibility that sensory input had an important part in the evoking process needed to be considered. Since seizures had been evoked by the sandpaper roughness discrimination test, the sandpaper blocks were rubbed over the surface of her fingers while her fingers were held quietly and passively at rest. Similarly the forms used in the TPT test were run through her fingers. These somatosensory stimuli evoked no dysrhythmia and no seizures.

The possibility still remained that position sense might be the evoking factor, therefore, the fingers of her right hand were manipulated for a prolonged period of time in the same manner as used in writing or finger tapping (Fig. 50). This did not evoke a seizure or EEG dysrhythmia.

Pinprick, light touch, and pinching the surface of her palms and fingers did not evoke a dysrhythmia. Visual input had no role. Blindfolding did not prevent the seizures from occurring (Fig. 51).

The foregoing studies rule out sensory input as a factor in the evocation of seizures. It appeared then that the movements themselves evoked the seizures. This left the possibility, however, that either the actual motion or the concept of motion might be the evoking factor. To study this, the patient's hand was placed on a finger tapping key. She was told not to press the key but to imagine that she was pressing it. There was continuous suggestion that she was feeling the motion of the key and hearing the click of the counter. There was no motion

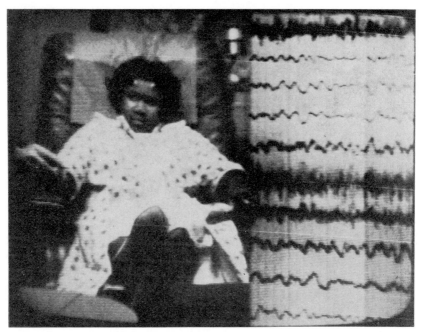

Figure 50.   Same patient. Sensory stimulation of right hand does not evoke seizures or dysrhythmia. Here index finger is being manipulated passively through the rate and range used in finger tapping.

of the fingers evident, and the key was not activated, nor could any muscle activity be detected by EMG. After several minutes of this suggestion, she had a typical seizure with the described dysrhythmia (Fig. 52). This was repeated several times, and the seizures were evoked, not by motor activity of sensory input, but only by the concept and mental imagery of motor activity.

The clinical picture of the episodes evoked by movement of a part of the body may be (a) choreoathetotic, (b) tonic, (c) clonic, (d) a combination of tonic and clonic, or (e) a major motor seizure. As noted previously, there has been some question of validity regarding the choreoathetotic form. Some authors feel this is primarily a disturbance of basal ganglia function. However, the choreoathetotic form, especially when it is associated with the significant EEG evoked dysrhythmia, must be considered as a form of reflex epilepsy. The reported tonic

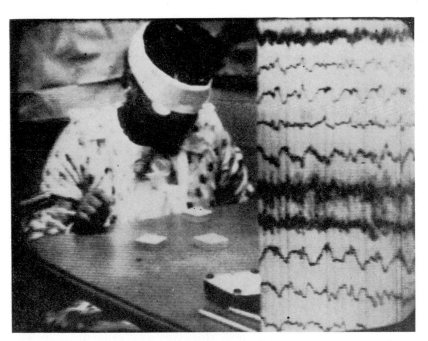

Figure 51. Same patient. Visual input has no role in seizure evocation. Here patient is blindfolded during sandpaper discrimination tests. Seizure evoked by manipulation of the blocks. Dysrhythmia as noted in Figures 48 and 49.

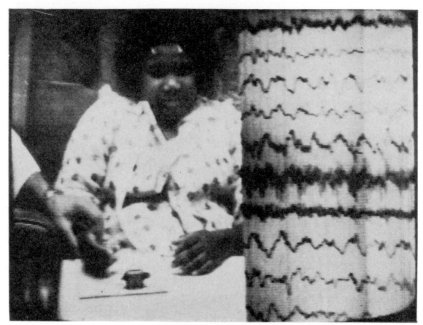

Figure 52.   Same patient.   Seizures evoked through suggestion of the concept of movement.   Dysrhythmia as in preceding figure.

forms, the clonic form (as in the study case, the case reported by Strauss,[13] and the evoked generalized seizure recorded by Pitha[12]) are definitely epileptic.

From both the study case and review of the literature, there appears to be wide variations as to the role of startle or suddenness in this form of reflex epilepsy. This is similar to the situation in auditory-evoked and in somatosensory-evoked seizures wherein startle varies in importance. While in many cases of movement-induced epilepsy in the literature, startle played a significant role, this did not happen in the Madison study patient. In some of the cases reported in the literature, the passive motion of an extremity in a startling fashion evoked seizures.

Strauss[13] emphasized the importance of the role of the motor component in his patient, and this was certainly true in the study subject as well. In the study patient, the possible evoking role of proprioceptive feedback and other sensory input has been ruled out. However, some of the reported incidences in the literature[8, 12] had seizures evoked by passive motion, thus inferring a sensory (especially a proprioceptive) factor.

In some of these patients, the seizures may be evoked by higher cognitive function, i.e. the thought of movement and the concept of motion. This has been demonstrated in the Research Laboratory. The case described by Pitha[12] had seizures evoked by watching an athlete run or even upon reading the report of a foot race. While the number of cases reported of seizures induced by movement is relatively small, wide variations are readily apparent in the nature of the evoking stimulus and type of seizure as well as in the possible role of the element of startle or surprise. The seizures may be evoked by sensory and especially proprioceptive stimuli or by the initiation or even the concept of initiation of movement. The seizures may be of various clinical types as noted above. The element of surprise or startle is necessary in some patients but does not play a role in seizure evocation in others.

REFERENCES

1. Gowers, W. R.: *Epilepsy*, London, 1901.
2. Lishman, W. A., Symonds, C. P., Whitty, C. W. M., and Willison, R. G.: Seizures induced by movement. *Brain*, 1962.
3. Burger, L. J., Lopez, R. E., and Elliott, F. A.: Tonic seizures induced by movement. *Neurology*, 22:656, 1972.
4. Loseau, P. and Marcombes: Motor seizures provoked by movement. *Bord Med*, 3:803, 1970.
5. Kurimoto, T., Kubota, S., and Kageyama, N.: Seizures induced by sudden start of voluntary movements. *J Kansai Med Sch*, 21:213, 1969.
6. Vranjesevic, D. and Radojicic, B.: Rare forms of epilepsy. *Neuropsihijatrija*, 19:155, 1971.
7. Fukyama, Y. and Okada, R.: Hereditary kinesthetic reflex epilepsy. *Proc Aust Assoc Neurol*, 5:583, 1968.
8. Gandiglio, G. and Gambi, D.: A case of epilepsy with both spontaneous and movement induced crises. *Rev Neurol*, 39:36, 1969.
9. Perez-Borja, C., Tassinari, A. C., and Swanson, A. G.: Paroxysmal choreoathetosis and seizures induced by movement. *Epilepsia*, 8:260, 1967.
10. Kato, M., Koga, M., Araki, S., and Kurowa, Y.: Kinetogenic seizures. Report of six cases. *Clin Neurol*, 10:299, 1970.

11. Michaux, L. and Granier, M.: Reflex Jacksonian epilepsy. *Ann Med Psychol, 103*:172, 1945.
12. Pitha, V.: Reflex epilepsy. *Rev Neurol, 70*:178-181, 1938.
13. Straus, H.: Jacksonian seizures of reflex origin. *Arch Neurol Psych, 44*:140, 1940.

CHAPTER 10

CLASSIFICATION OF REFLEX EPILEPSY

IN THE PRECEDING chapters, seventy-three instances of evoked epilepsy were presented, and the pertinent literature was discussed. It is obvious that wide differences exist among the cases of reflex epilepsy both in regard to kinds of stimuli and in stimulus response. In 1972,[1] the author devised a classification of reflex epilepsy based on these differences. Subsequent observations in the laboratory permit new and more extensive deductions regarding the differences, and Table XI presents the differences in stimuli and stimulus responses between the simple, or primary, and the complex, or secondary, types of reflex epilepsy.

The evoking stimuli differ considerably between the two types. In the simple type, the evoking stimulus is easily definable and simple; for example, a sudden, loud, nonspecific noise, a flickering light, a specific visual pattern, a brisk, unexpected tap, or a startling passive motion to a particular part of the body.

TABLE XI

BASIS FOR CLASSIFICATION OF REFLEX EPILEPSY
TYPES OF REFLEX EPILEPSY

	SIMPLE	COMPLEX
Stimulus characteristic	Simple	Complex
Stimulus intensity	Important	Not important
Stimulus-response time	Immediate	Delayed
Unilateral stimulus presentation	Nonevoking	Evoking
Stimulus presentation during sleep	Nonevoking	Evoking
Evoked dysrhythmia	Generalized	Focal cortical
Evoked seizures	Generalized	Focal
Mixed seizures	Within type	Within type
Postictal refractory period	None	Present
Medications most likely to alter response	Benzodiazepines	Hydantoinates, primidone

By constrast, in the complex type of reflex epilepsy, the stimulus is more difficult to define. The stimulus here may consist of, for example, the theme of music, the acquisition or communication of knowledge in language epilepsy, decision making in the patient with seizures playing chess, the imagined concept of movement of a body part, or the elusive characteristics of the evoking stimulus such as was described in the patients with eating epilepsy.

Significant differences occur between the two types with respect to stimulus intensity. In the simple type, the intensity is important, as was noted in photosensitivity where the intensity had to be determined for the individual patient. (For example, patterns presented in dim ambient light do not evoke dysrhythmias.) By contrast in the complex type, stimulus intensity plays a much less important role. In musicogenic epilepsy, sound levels are not important, and the music need not even be consciously perceived. Intensity is of course difficult to evaluate in reading epilepsy, but when the reading material is legible, it evokes seizures. In decision-making epilepsy, it is difficult to quantitate stimulus intensity.

There is a marked difference between the two types with regard to stimulus-response time. The appearance of the abnormal responses varies considerably in its temporal relationship to the presentation of the stimuli. In the simple types of reflex epilepsy, the response is usually immediate or very nearly immediate with the presentation of the appropriate stimulus. The flicker flash or the sudden noise usually evokes a seizure within a fraction of a second. But in the complex type, the stimulus needs to be applied for a period of time. For example, in musicogenic epilepsy, this may vary up to several minutes and in reading epilepsy may require hours. It is even noteworthy that the stimulus-response time varies in the same patient in the complex type, as shown most dramatically in the case of eating epilepsy. (The variations also occurred in the cases of musicogenic epilepsy and in the patients with reading epilepsy.)

An important observation in the laboratories has been the result of unilateral presentation of the evoking stimulus in reflex epilepsy. This has been noted previously by the author and his colleagues in relationship to photosensitivity[2, 3] and to acoustico-motor epilepsy[4] and has been considered in a separate short publication.[5] The particular caution needed in determining the effect of unilateral presentation of the stimulus has also been discussed in the photosensitive patient. It is important to occlude completely the vision of one eye, and in the auditory-evoked, startle, or acousticomotor epilepsy, it was noted that the sound level has to be kept below 60 decibels to prevent bone conduction to the opposite ear and thus an inadvertant binaural stimulation. In the cases of simple reflex epilepsy, unilateral presentations usually fail to evoke a seizure. This is not universal but very nearly so as indicated in the survey of the study patients with photosensitive, pattern, and eye closure seizures. By contrast, however, in the complex types of reflex epilepsy, unilateral presentation, when relevant, inevitably evokes the seizures. This occurred in all study cases of reading epilepsy, in the patient who experienced seizures with decision making, and in the musicogenic patients. It also occurred in the patient with color/object-induced epilepsy.

Presentation of the evoking stimulus during sleep in the simple type of reflex epilepsy usually fails to evoke a seizure. This has been noted n the Research Laboratory and by others[6] in patients with photosensitivity. However, in the complex type of reflex epilepsy, presentation of the appropriate stimulus during sleep evokes a seizure. This has been demonstrated by the study in musicogenic epilepsy and in voice-induced epilepsy. It cannot be studied in reading epilepsy nor in eating epilepsy because the very nature of the evoking stimulus precludes its presentation in the sleep state.

At present the laboratory has not gained sufficient data, nor have the author and his colleagues much intent to pursue the point, but it appears that the responses during sleep are similar to those obtained in patients under hypnosis, with hypnotic suggestion replacing the evoking stimulus. In one patient with photosensitivity, hypnotic suggestion of the presentation of the evoking stimulus at the proper flicker frequency failed to evoke a seizure. But in the patient with voice-induced epilepsy and in one of the musicogenic patients, seizures occurred on the suggestion that the appropriate stimulus was being presented. Also, in the patient with movement-induced epilepsy, the suggestion of movement (without the actual initiation of movement) induced seizures. These are not sufficient observations to permit definite conclusions, but they indicate that the mental concept of the evoking stimulus suffices to evoke a seizure in many of the patients with the complex forms of reflex epilepsy. The laboratory maintains little interest in hypnosis and has not uniformly employed it in the study patients; it was used only for special purposes in these particular patients.

The evoked electroencephalographic dysrhythmia is also quite different between these two types of reflex epilepsy. In the simple type, the dysrhythmia is primarily generalized, i.e. a centrencephalic type of dysrhythmia although often of the atypical wave and spike form. The reticular formation of the centrencephalic system as proposed by Penfield is involved either in primary or secondary fashion. In the complex types of reflex epilepsy, the electroencephalographic abnormalities are primarily focal cortical, as in the patients with musicogenic epilepsy, in the seizures evoked by eating or movement, in the patient with voice-induced epilepsy, and in reading epilepsies.

The clinical types of seizures are also different. In the simple type of reflex epilepsy, the seizure type is often generalized, frequently of the absence or myoclonic type and occasionally generalized major motor. By contrast, in the complex type of reflex epilepsy, the seizures are usually focal—for example, temporal lobe automatisms in musicogenic epilepsy, or aphasic seizures in voice-induced epilepsy, and seizures of paralysis in eating epilepsy.

The specificity of the seizures in the higher cognitive functions—communication seizures or language/reading—is especially significant. Here the motor manifestation of the seizure varies with the expression of communication. Jaw jerk and vocalization occurred when reading aloud, but tonic or clonic seizures of the hand occurred with manual communication as in writing, in playing the piano, or in transcribing notes. While major motor seizures may occur in either the simple or complex types, they are probably more common in the simple type.

Mixed evoked seizure types occur. This has been previously noted in the visually induced forms of seizures where patients had combinations of photic, pattern, and eye closure seizures. Also, combinations of forms of simple epilepsy occur. For example, in Chapter 3 it was noted that Case 4 (with auditory-evoked epilepsy) also had some somatosensory-evoked seizures. Some patients may have startle-induced seizures evoked by light, sound, or somatosensory stimuli.

The combinations in the complex type have also been described. For example, in reading epilepsy, Case 4 also had seizures while singing, and the reading epilepsy Case 9 had evoked dysrhythmia while engaging in problems of decision making. The study did not examine any patient with mixed seizure types including both the simple and complex forms. There are, however, in the literature isolated suggestions of this. An example is the patient described as having photosensitivity and reading epilepsy.[7] However, the author was unable to evoke reading epilepsy in the laboratory, and the response to photic stimulation was of the driving type followed later by a single sharp wave. The rarity with which mixed seizures occur between the two types of reflex epilepsy indicates that mixed seizure forms tend to occur within the type of simple or complex reflex epilepsy and rarely if ever cross this boundary.

A significant difference is present between the two types in the occurrences of a postictal refractory period. Repeated presentation of the evoking stimulus in the patients with the simple type of reflex epilepsy produces repeated seizures. If a patient with photosensitivity has a flicker-evoked seizure and the stroboscopic stimulation is continued (Fig. 53), after a period of time a subsequent seizure will occur. By contrast, in the complex type, repeated presentation will not evoke a second seizure. For example, if in musicogenic epilepsy the evoking music is continued through the clinical seizure and the postictal period of confusion, during which the EEG slowing occurs, and is further continued into the normal state, both clinically and electroencephalographically, no seizure occurs. Noted in the chapter on somatosensory epilepsy was the effect of the refractory

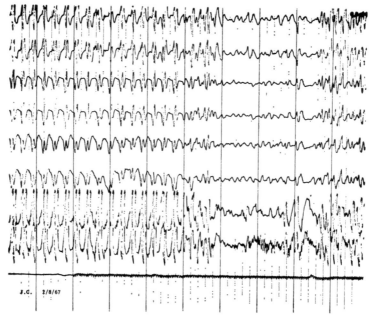

Figure 53.   Continuous photic stimulation during and after photic-induced seizure discharge. Recurrence of evoked dysrhythmia indicates there is no postictal refractory period in the simple type of reflex epilepsy. Bottom channel records strobe stimulations.

period in Case 4. This phenomenon interfered with the study until it was appreciated as such.

Certain pharmacological differences also seem to exist between the two types in that patients with the simple type of reflex epilepsy may respond to diazepam derivatives whereas some of the complex types of reflex epilepsy (e.g. decision-making and movement-induced) may respond to the more traditional hydantoin and primidone types of medication. In general, however, the response to medication in both types leaves much to be desired. This is discussed at greater length in Chapter 14.

Based upon these classification criteria, the cases studied in the Epilepsy Research Laboratory and those in the literature can be divided into the simple and complex types. It should be noted that, as in all clinical research, not every patient will fit each and every point in the criteria. Some criteria are *de facto* impossible to fulfill; for example, acousticomotor responses occur only in the waking state because the acoustic stimulus wakes the patient. Also, in some somatosensory-evoked epilepsy (as in Cases 1 and 2), unilateral presentations were necessary to evoke the seizures because of the nature of the reflexogenous zone.

Presentations during sleep are obviously impossible in reading epilepsy. In the patients whose evoking stimuli lie within their own control, repeated presentations are not possible since the patient must administer the stimulus. An example of this is the case of eating epilepsy. With ictal and postictal paralysis of pharynx, larynx, and tongue, no presentation was possible during the refractory period, for the patient could not eat. Taking into account these factors in real life constraints, it is still possible to arrive at a reasonable classification (Table XII).

The classification in Table XII is based largely on the case observations in the Research Laboratory. The entries in parentheses are cases reported by others and of forms not directly

TABLE XII

CLASSIFICATION OF REFLEX EPILEPSY

	SIMPLE TYPE	COMPLEX TYPE
Visually induced Reflex epilepsy	Photosensitivity Pattern-evoked Eye-closure induced	Color-induced
Auditory-evoked Reflex epilepsy	Evoked by nonspecific startling sounds	Specific but nonverbal sounds without startle Specific voices
Musicogenic	(Musicogenic—certain notes)	Musicogenic evoked by themes
Movement-induced	(Evoked by startling passive movement)	Evoked by active movement or concept of movement
Communications/reading epilepsy	(Due to eye movement, or patterns)	Due to acquisition of knowledge
Decision-making		Sequential decision making under stress
Somtosensory-evoked epilepsy	Evoked by startling tap stimulation	Evoked by prolonged nonstartle stimulation
Seizures related to eating	(Myoclonic attacks with swallowing)	With eating, but obscure evoking stimulus

(   ) Cases cited from literature and not studied in the laboratory.

studied in the laboratory. For example, in none of the study's reading epileptics did eye or jaw movement or the pattern of the printed page play a role. The entries in parentheses are for the documented cases where they did play a role, as explained in Chapter 6. In musicogenic epilepsy, the evoking stimulus in the study's five patients was subtle and resided in the theme of the music. In the case of Poskanzer et al.[8] however, it was clearly shown that the evoking stimulus was a certain musical note. The case of eating epilepsy with myoclonic attacks on swallowing was described by Stevens in the discussion of the present author's paper.[9]

An important fact to be derived from Table XII is that reflex epilepsies occurring in response to certain stimuli need not be of the same type. For example, all reading epilepsies are not of the complex type. The same is true of musicogenic epilepsy, the auditory-evoked epilepsies in general, and in visually induced seizures. It is obvious from reviewing Table XII that merely because seizures occur with a particular kind of stimulus (visual, auditory, language, etc.), the case does not immediately fall into the simple or complex type of reflex epilepsy. The inference is that *careful standardized studies are necessary to determine in each case whether or not the stimulus evoked epilepsy is simple or complex.* For example, in the musicogenic epileptic patient it is necessary to determine whether the stimulus is a theme of music or a particular note and in the reading epilepsy, whether it is eye movement or patterns rather than the acquisition of knowledge.

One might question placing the color/object-induced epilepsy in the complex type, especially since the laboratory studies were limited by the subject's hyperactivity and mental retardation. However, this youngster was monocularly sensitive, the stimuli (the color red or viewing his hand) were complex, the seizures did not appear immediately but might require a minute or more after he hunched over the object, and the seizures became progressively less severe during a prolonged period of stimulation. The first seizure after a long seizure-free period, for example in the morning, would be a rather severe tonic seizure, and continuing stimulation would evoke myoclonic jerks of decreasing severity until he became refractory. For these reasons, his case belongs in the complex group.

The difference between the simple and complex types of reflex epilepsy suggests different neurophysiological mechanisms. In the simple type, the nature and type of stimulus, the quick response, and the probable involvement of centrencephalic structures suggest involvement of primary receptor cortex and/or subcortical structures. The studies in some acousticomotor seizures, using Anectine to block the myoclonic movement, demonstrated the absence of significant EEG abnormality upon presentation of the stimulus. Thus it is evident that subcortical mechanisms only may be involved in some of the patients, while in others the cerebral cortex may be the primary receptive central nervous system area for the particular stimulus, with subsequent centrencephalic involvement.

By contrast, in the complex type of reflex epilepsy, the complex nature of the stimulus, the delayed response to the stimulus, and in some cases the types of seizures evoked, suggest that supplementary and association areas of cortex may be the regions from which the seizure discharges are evoked.

One might postulate from these observations that the simple type of reflex epilepesy can be evidenced at a lower or less developed region of the nervous system. The simplicity of stimulus and response in the patients and the fact that these types of reflex epilepsy can be induced in animals (Chapter 16) suggest that the regions of the nervous system involved in the simple types of reflex epilepsy are at lower levels. This is further supported by the fact that in some of these forms (e.g. acoustico-motor) the attacks may be subcortical (as shown by the Anectine studies) or dependent upon impaired inhibition.

Moreover, the simple type of reflex epilepsy can occur with degenerative or widespread disease of the nervous system. Photosensitivity has been demonstrated in patients with cerebellar degeneration and multiple sclerosis. The simple type also occurs in patients with partially developed brains, for example the study case with trisomy-D anomaly (alobar prosencephaly). But the complex types, dependent as they are on higher nervous system functions, are not seen with failure of maturation or subsequent widespread severe destruction of the central nervous system.

By contrast, the complex forms are dependent upon higher nervous system functions, for example the discrimination of certain themes of music, the communication of ideas, either afferent or efferent, or even the complexities of decision making. Moreover it has been shown that memory (in musicogenic epilepsy), anticipation (in eating epilepsy), and the concept of the evoking stimulum (movement-induced epilepsy) may play a role in such seizure evocation. Suggestion, simple or hypnotic, can induce the seizures in at least some instances of the complex type. Obviously then, the complex types of reflex epilepsy are related to higher nervous system functions, especially those involving association areas of cortex and their connections.

REFERENCES

1. Forster, F. M.: The classification and conditioning treatment of the reflex epilepsies. *Int J Neurol, 9*:73, 1972.
2. Forster, F. M. and Campos, G. B.: Conditioning factors in stroboscopic-induced seizures. *Epilepsia, 5*:156, 1964.
3. Forster, F. M., Ptacek, L. J., Peterson, W. G., Chun, R. W. M., Bengzon, A. R. A., and Campos, G. B.: Strobscopic-induced seizure discharge. *Arch Neurol, 11*:603, 1964.
4. Booker, H. E., Forster, F. M., and Klove, H.: Extinction factors in startle (acoustico-motor) seizures. *Neurology, 15*:1095, 1965.
5. Forster, F. M.: Unilateral special sensory stimulation in sensory evoked epilepsy. *Trans VI Int Cong of EEG and Clin Neurophy* Vienna, 53-60, September, 1965.
6. Scollo-Lavizzari, G. and Hess, R.: Photic stimulation during paradoxical sleep in photosensitive patients. *Neurology, 17*:604, 1967.
7. Blumenthal, I. J. and Dunn, A. T.: Reading epilepsy combined with intermittent photic stimulation: Case report. *Psychosom Med, 134*:85, 1966.
8. Poskanzer, C., Brown, E., and Miller, H.: Musicogenic epilepsy caused only by a discrete frequency band of church bells. *Brain, 85*:77, 1962.
9. Stevens, H., in discussion of Forster, F. M.: Epilepsy associated with eating. *Trans Am Neurol Assoc, 96*:106, 1971.

CHAPTER 11

DIFFERENTIAL DIAGNOSIS OF
REFLEX EPILEPSY

IT WOULD SEEM that the diagnosis of reflex epilepsy, that is, the administration of the given stimulus and the evocation of seizures, might be relatively simple. In Chapter 1, however, mention was made of the need to establish that a definite or presumed seizure in a given patient was in fact evoked by a specific stimulus. Most of the patients with reflex epilepsy whose cases are reported in this book were referred for evaluation or therapy, often from a considerable distance. Others were selected from the patient population group of the Neurology Clinic. However, not all the patients studied by the described methods had reflex epilepsy, nor indeed did they all have epilepsy. In this chapter, various entities which closely mimic the reflex epilepsies are discussed.

CHANCE OCCURRENCE OF SEIZURES UPON
STIMULUS PRESENTATION

A number of patients referred for "reflex epilepsy" definitely had epilepsy. Also, some of their seizures occurred when they were presented with evoking stimuli. However, the inconsistency of the stimulus response and the high incidence of spontaneous seizures eliminated these patients as potential cases of reflex epilepsy. Examples of this were patients with frequent petit mal seizures and inconsistent responses when exposed to the standard methods of testing. These patients might show a dysrhythmia on exposure to a particular pattern on the first series of tests, to no pattern on the second series, and to yet a different pattern on the third test. These patients were not considered to have pattern-evoked epilepsy. The inconsistent evocation of the dysrhythmia might also occur with monocular presentations, adding further confirmation to the opinion that the seizures and dysrhythmia were coincidental and not related to the stimulus.

The chance occurrence of seizures during stimulus presentation may also happen in the complex type of reflex epilepsy. Also studied was a twenty-year-old student who had frequent psychomotor seizures, some of which had occurred while listening to music. On two consecutive days, he was monitored with AV tape recordings while he listened for a total of eight hours to the full range of music used in the laboratory. While occasional theta activity occurred in the left temporal region, this was not associated with symptoms and did not recur when the same musical number was replayed or when similar musical numbers were played. This alteration of the EEG also occurred in the resting record and when recorded during sensory deprivation. This study demonstrated that the mere occurrence of a dysrhythmia or seizure while listening to music does not constitute musicogenic epilepsy.

Another patient was referred as a possible case of epilepsy evoked by eating. This patient had psychomotor seizures when eating but also had them at other times. It was found that they occurred during sensory deprivation, in the resting state, during the neurological examination, while in the elevator on the way to the laboratory, and of course while eating. The seizures which occurred while eating were merely chance or nonspecific occurrences.

NONEPILEPTIC STIMULUS RESPONSES

In ten patients, the study found a consistent stimulus response to a particular sensory stimulation. The clinical responses, however, were certainly not reflex epilepsy (indeed, were not even epileptic) and were not associated with a cerebral dysrhythmia.

The occurrence of symptoms or a syndrome which might potentially be confused with reflex epilepsy occurred preponderantly in relationship to the complex type of reflex epilepsy. Of the seventy-three patients with reflex epilepsy reported in this volume, forty-nine had the simple type of reflex epilepsy. Only three patients presented a syndrome mimicking to some extent simple reflex epilepsy. By contrast, there were twenty-two cases of the complex type of reflex epilepsy and seven diagnostically confusing syndroms. This disproportion is significant but not surprising. Many of the complex types of reflex epilepsy are related to higher cognitive functions, and while skillful testing is necessary in all forms of reflex epilepsy, the diagnostic evaluation must be especially searching in the complex type because of the complexity of the stimulus and the variability of the stimulus-response interval.

Hyperventilation Syndrome

Three patients presented with hyperventilation syndromes evoked by the stimulus presentation. In two of these patients (Cases 1 and 2) the stimulus presentation was visual, and in one, musical (Case 3).

CASE 1. This patient was suspected of having photosensitive seizures but had a neurotic anxiety reaction with hyperventilation induced by stroboscopic stimulation and unaccompanied by EEG dysrhythmia. This patient, a twenty-five-year-old female, noticed over the past four years that lights bothered her. They seemed to be too bright, and she was especialy bothered by glare from shiny walls and flooring. She noticed that the glare became flashing and seemed to have a sparkling element which especially frightened her. She was unable to tolerate the sensations she experienced when exposed to flashing lights from glaring walls or ceilings, and for this reason, she dropped out of school.

The patient reported a typical episode as follows: She would notice that contrasts between colors became particularly intense and that objects lost their three-dimensionality. She had difficulty with depth perception. In approximately half of these episodes, she noticed that her hands became numb and tingling. She felt panicky, cried profusely, and was afraid to be alone. The episodes were reported as lasting ten to fifteen minutes.

The patient described herself as a chronic hypochondriac as a child. She stated that between the ages of twelve and fourteen she had several episodes of severe migraine headaches, beginning with flashing lights, which progressed to near-blindness. Her last such headache occurred when she was twenty-three years old. Also as a child she had several episodes of prolonged, severe abdominal cramping which lasted up to seven hours.

The physical and neurological examinations were negative.

When studied in the Epilepsy Research Laboratory, she was exposed to stroboscopic stimulations, eyes open and closed, binocularly and monocularly, from one flash per second to flicker fusion point. At no time were dysrhythmias elicited. However, when the stimulations were in the fifteen to twenty cycles per second range, she felt very uncomfortable. The discomfort was more severe with eyes open than with eyes closed. Prolonged stimulations within this range evoked hyperventilation, crying out, a feeling of being "drawn in," followed by numbness of the hands. This occurred with both monocular and binocular stimulation.

Upon presentations of visual patterns no dysrhythmia was evoked. Since some of her episodes occurred in places of modern entertainment (discotheques), stroboscopic stimulation was coupled with the type of music presented in these entertainment places. The combination of music and photic stimulation did not evoke dysrhythmia or seizures. The episodes obtained by photic stimulation were reproducible over a three-day period when she was studied in the laboratory, and when carried on for a sufficient period of time, these anxiety states proceeded into a hyperventilation syndrome.

CASE 2. This patient also presented a hyperventilation syndrome, but in this instance it was evoked by viewing certain patterns. The patient also definitely had psychomotor seizures, but these were not related to sensory stimulation.

She was a sixteen-year-old girl who was known to have had seizures since the age of six. During these episodes she lost awareness of all events for several minutes. She described episodes in which she would be walking inside the school building and would suddenly find herself in a different part of the school. She could not remember walking to this area but she deduced that it must have taken her at least three or four minutes to arrive there. These episodes also occurred when driving a car;

she found herself in a strange part of town without knowledge of how she arrived there. The patient had been told by a friend that she licked her lips prior to the beginning of these episodes. The episodes were followed by a period of amnesia lasting from five to twenty-five minutes.

Her parents felt that she had seizures in particular parts of the house (in the bathroom and in her bedroom) and that these were evoked by certain visual patterns in these rooms.

The past medical history and family history were negative, as were physical and neurological examinations.

All laboratory tests were normal except a sleep EEG which showed the presence of an epileptogenic focus in the right anterior temporal lobe. She was studied in the Epilepsy Research Laboratory for the possibility of visually induced seizures and was presented with the usual stroboscopic stimulations. These studies were negative. She was presented with the usual gamut of patterns, and there was no indication of visually evoked seizures or dysrhythmia.

Her father brought to the laboratory a shag rug from her bathroom which was reported to have evoked seizures and also samples of wallpaper from her bedroom. These were presented to her and she stared at them approximately one minute. This presentation evoked a bizarre clinical response characterized by stiffening of the body and tightening of the fingers and jaw muscles. Hyperventilation occurred to the point of a positive Chvostek sign. There was no loss of consciousness since she could be induced to talk during these episodes. At no time was there any EEG change associated with these stimulus presentations. During her course in the hospital, the patient had several classical psychomotor seizures not related to any particular visual stimulus. The patient therefore had classical psychomotor epilepsy, but there was no indication of reflex epilepsy. She did, however, have a pattern-induced hyperventilation syndrome.

CASE 3. This thirty-nine-year-old female had a hyperventilation syndrome evoked by music. For approximately six years she noticed that music made her feel uncomfortable, and she began having attacks in which her respirations became rapid and she would lose consciousness. She injured herself several times in these episodes. No specific type of music was implicated, but jangling, fast, echo-chamber type of music (with guitars) and other shrill music were thought to be the most likely to stimulate these episodes. Because of these episodes of loss of consciousness she had been diagnosed as having musicogenic epilepsy and had been treated with anticonvulsant medications.

The physical and neurological examinations were normal, as were the laboratory studies.

She was studied for a two-week period in the Research Laboratory. She was exposed to various types of music, and it was noted that Rock and Roll and guitar types of music readily induced hyperventilation with tossing of the head from side to side. The hyperventilation proceeded to the point of a positive Chvostek's sign and sometimes to the point of unconsciousness. During this time the EEG showed only artifacts consistent with her eye blinks and head movement, but at no time were there any evoked dysrhythmias.

During the course of her studies it was learned that her husband owned a music store in which she had to work part-time, and she was not pleased with this occupation. Thus there was an obvious secondary gain, for the hyperventilation syndrome precluded working in the store.

Syncope

Case 4.   This patient was an example of vasovagal syncope evoked by visual stimuli. This twenty-five-year-old sophomore medical student was referred because of a witnessed "seizure." While observing a patient with severe body burns during a class in physical diagnosis, he lost consciousness and had some twitching movements. The physician who witnessed the episode thought it was convulsive. On questioning, it developed that he had had a series of some six similar episodes, each precipitated by some subjective or objective health-related episode. These episodes began with the reception of inoculations at the age of twelve years and had occurred while watching medical movies. His only significant illness was severe pneumonia in infancy. There was no history of any seizure manifestations other than noted above. There was no history of convulsive disorders in his family. Physical and neurological examinations were normal.

He was sent for an EEG, and when the last electrodes were being filled with saline, he had a similar episode. The technician then began to run the EEG and marked slowing, considered at first to be postictal slowing, was noted. To determine if the patient had seizures evoked by viewing unpleasant sights, he was monitored in the laboratory. His EKG was continuously recorded on one channel of the EEG machine, his EEGs on the other fifteen channels. He was presented with an American College of Surgeons film. This film, demonstrating rectal resection by the abdominal and perineal routes, was espeically chosen for its vivid depiction.

After some six minutes of viewing the film, he attempted to turn his head away, but was told to continue looking. He did so. His heart rate dropped gradually from eighty-six per minute to forty-two. He became pale, slumped forward in the chair, and had a few generalized twitching movements. His EEG became very slow, and high voltage in all leads (but no epileptogenic discharges occurred). When he was placed in the recumbent position, his heart rate returned to normal and so did his EEG.

This patient had a vasovagal syncope, evoked by viewing "horrible sights." Reference is made to this in Chapter 2.

Pseudoseizures

CASE 5. This was the only patient who had pseudoseizures evoked by the appropriate stimulus. The sixteen-year-old, male high school graduate was referred for evaluation of possible musicogenic epilepsy. His first seizure occurred when he was twelve years of age, while attending a junior high school band concert. His seizures occurred after listening to modern guitar music. According to him, the seizures continued as long as the music did and would disappear when the music stopped. In junior high school, his classmates discovered his difficulties and teased him by playing the offending music. On occasions he would be exposed to music in educational movies and would have a seizure. He was told that each seizure lasted from one to fifteen minutes. He allegedly had tonic and clonic movements, regained consciousness immediately after the end of the music, and complained of being tired afterwards. He had been taking multiple kinds of anticonvulsant medications.

He consistently carried with him two electronic mechanical devices. One of these was a small, battery-operated tape recorder loaded with classical music, and the other a white noise generator. Either could be played through the stereo earphones which he wore constantly in order to block out the possibility of any exposure to the particular types of music which he perceived as noxious.

The family history was negative. The physical and neurological examinations and laboratory data were all normal, as were hearing tests.

In the Epilepsy Research Laboratory he was exposed to various kinds of taped music. At the first sound of electric guitar music, he had what he later stated was a "typical attack."

The seizures always occurred upon his immediate awareness of electric guitar music, consisted of tonic stiffening of all four extremities and neck with some rhythmic movements, which, judging by their appearance and especially by the muscle artifact in the EEG, were synchronized to the beat in the music. This persisted as long as the music was played. He claimed that during this period he did not know what was transpiring and that he was in a "grey area." During the "seizures" evoked by playing of the music, his extremities could be molded into position and were held in uncomfortable and awkward positions, such as tonic extension, without support for the duration of the musical number (on one occasion for as long as twenty-four minutes). He stated that he was aware that his arms were held up when he "came to," but had no idea how they had gotten into that position. There was no postictal confusion and no postictal refractory period, for another episode could be induced within seconds.

During some fifteen hours of recording in the laboratory, no EEG abnormality was noted. This included resting records, recording during sleep, and recording during the exposure to music, for the periods before, during, and after the seizures. Neither dysrhythmia nor postictal slowing occurred.

Guitar music was presented through stereophonic earphones, first into the right ear only, and then into the left ear only. The sound was kept at a level well below 60 decibels so as not to allow bone conduction to the opposite ear. He rather liked this music, thought it was "boogie woogie," and was not aware of the sound of the electric guitar. This was played then into both ears, and as the volume was increased, he recognized the electric guitar and had a "seizure."

He was also studied during sleep. Sleep was induced by sleep deprivation and chloral hydrate. In stage IV sleep, the guitar music was played very softly and gradually increased. No seizure occurred, even though it was played much louder than in the waking state. He was called, touched, and awakened while the music was being played; he then had a "seizure."

For these episodes to occur awareness on his part of the sound of the electric guitar was needed, and yet, as noted on the playback of the AV tape recordings on at least one occasion, using a musical number which had evoked a previous seizure, the seizurelike episode occurred prior to the introduction of the electric guitar when he anticipated the introduction.

These episodes were considered to be evoked pseudoseizures in view of the following facts: (a) the "seizures" were atypical, (b) there were no EEG concomitants of epileptiform discharges, (c) no postictal confusion, and (d) no postictal slowing occurred.

The attacks were also atypical for musicogenic epilepsy in that they were not evoked by monaural stimulations until it was recognized via binaural stimulation that the electric guitar was present, and they were not evoked while asleep. Also, the repeated playing of a particular noxious number did not render it innocuous as occurs in bona fide musicogenic epilepsy. Playing a particular noxious number for approximately twenty-four minutes led to no cessation of the tonic contractions. Instead the rhythmic movements became considerably more exaggerated, and there was no indication of decrease in the pseudoseizure clinical activity.

Episodic Midbrain Dysfunction

CASE 6. This patient had an episodic midbrain dysfunction of unknown etiology which was initially confused with photosensitivity. A forty-four-year-old mother of four, she had a two-day episode of "imbalance" at age twenty-four, with some recurrence ten years later. This was diagnosed as labyrinthitis. The patient was well until age thirty-nine, when she experienced the insidious onset of an episodic lightheaded feeling, and easily evoked irritability. She began to notice nausea with reading. Some nystagmus was noted about that time. Several months later the patient became weak, ataxic, lethargic, and quite ill. She was hospitalized, and EEG, skull X ray, and cerebrospinal fluid studies were normal. She improved somewhat, but then gradually became worse. Two years later she became acutely ill with severe lethargy, balance disorder, giddiness, and some nausea, all of which tended to be episodic in nature, but with a constant underlying discomfort. Spontaneous bilateral nystagmus was then documented.

During the ensuing year the patient's episodes of dizziness and lethargy became worse, and she noted weakness in right upper and lower extremities. A right lower facial nerve weakness was noted. ENT evaluations and caloric evaluations were normal.

At age forty-one, she developed transient double vision and mild bilateral weakness of the lateral rectus muscles. At that time she had the first attack which included marked stupor (from which the patient was arousable with vigorous stimulation), marked nystagmus, partial right sixth nerve palsy, and marked ataxia. An EEG during the attack was reportedly normal. Brain scan, skull films, and right retrobrachial arteriograms were also normal.

The patient subsequently continued to have "attacks," many of which were precipitated by such visual stimuli as flickering lights, moderate reading, or eye scanning activity. These episodes lasted from a few seconds to several minutes, and frequently were noted to include marked stupor, left sixth nerve paresis, hemiparesis of the right side, left facial palsy, and severe left maxillary and suborbital pain. Lip smacking movements were occasionally noted.

A pneumoencephalogram performed elsewhere was reportedly normal, and a course of adrenocorticotropic hormone (ACTH) therapy was instituted without benefit. Medications at the time of admission included: carbamazepine 400 mg four times a day, Thorazine® 25 mg by mouth as needed for control of nausea, amphetamines 15 to 25 mg as needed to treat the stupor, Premarin® 1.25 mg daily for menstrual irregularity, Diuril® 500 mg as needed to treat premenstrual edema, Percodan® as needed for facial pain (used rarely), and Valium® which was used occasionally for sleep. The patient reported that alcohol and barbiturates greatly exacerbated her symptoms.

Past medical history was negative. Family history revealed the patient's father died at age seventy-five of a frontal lobe tumor. On physical examination she was presented as an obese, forty-four-year-old white woman wearing a patch over the left eye and in no acute distress. Shortly after admission the patient had a forty-five-second attack characterized by stupor, slurred speech, flickering eyelids, dysconjugate eye movements, and marked quivering of the left lower lip. Marked strabismus of the left eye was also noted during the attack. The attacks were precipitated by ophthalmoscopic examination and testing of the extraocular movements. Cranial nerves were intact. Motor strength was good. All sensory modalities were intact. Cerebellar functions were good except for an abnormal gait with forward and backward pitching of the body at times. Reflexes were normal.

Laboratory and X-ray data were negative except that serum immunoelectrophoresis showed marked decrease of all immunoglobulin, especially IgA IgM. Chest X ray, skull X rays, and tomograms of the internal auditory canals were normal. The outside arteriograms and pneumoencephalgram were reviewed and felt to be normal. Neuropsychological testing showed no evidence of adaptive or cognitive impairment.

In the laboratory, various stimuli evoked a definite clinical response, unaccompanied by EEG changes. The clinical responses consisted of episodes of slurring of speech, ataxic gait, and twitching of the face; the most marked feature was a convergence spasm of the eyes. These episodes lasted from one to five minutes.

The clinical response could be evoked by stroboscopic stimulation, by reading, or by eye movement. A visual component was not necessary to induce the episodes. When the patient's eyes were held closed, her hand was moved from side to side, and she was instructed to follow her index finger with her eyes, episodes could be readily elicited.

This patient was felt to have a paroxysmal midbrain disorder evoked by multiple stimuli, not epileptic in nature and of obscure etiology. Her previous therapeutic regimens indicate that her neurologists had entertained at times the possibility of an epileptic disorder and at other times a demyelinizing disease.

Autonomic Disturbance

CASE 7. This patient was referred for evaluation of a peculiar depressed feeling when listening to music, and the question was raised if at these times he was having minor. seizures. The evaluation revealed no seizure disturbance but instead a loss of autonomic responses to music.

The patient was a forty-nine-year-old male with a masters degree in music. He had served as a music critic for some years. While he was well trained in the technical and intellectual aspects of music, he also enjoyed music because it "did something for me emotionally." Fifteen months before the time of the study, the patient suffered a spontaneous subarachnoid hemorrhage. Carotid angiography demonstrated an aneurysm in the right middle cerebral artery, and intracranial surgery was performed. Three weeks after this surgery, a small extradural hematoma was drained through a burr hole.

The patient's recovery was uneventful, although he began to notice some peculiar distortions of his perception. Music sounded off key, flat, and monotonous. Music did not evoke in him any of the previous usual pleasurable emotions. He was able to read musical scores and to play the piano, although this was done quite slowly and laboriously. He experienced the same difficulty in reading scores whether he was playing the piano or not. He had never been a particularly good singer. However, he noted that he constantly sang off key but was unable to correct it. In addition, peoples' faces, especially their eyes, seemed to look alike to him. Peoples' voices seem to have no inflections, and he felt that his own voice and other peoples' voices all tended to sound alike. The changes in his response to music were so marked that he found it necessary to stop listening to his extensive record library of classical music. Previously, this had been a major avocation. With the passage of time, these symptoms began to be associated with more generalized feelings of depression.

At the time of the study, the general physical examination was unremarkable, and the neurologic examination revealed only mild weakness of left hand grip. He obtained a Verbal IQ of 123 and a Performance IQ of 99 on the Wechsler Adult Intelligence Scale, a split compatible with right hemisphere dysfunction. Skull X rays showed the operative defects. An electroencephalogram showed some four- to seven-cycle-per-second theta activity in the right sylvian parietal region, with sharp contoured waves in the same area. Listening to music of different kinds did not significantly change his electroencephalograms.

He was able to recognize the music played for him, and was able to accurately criticize technique and performance. On the Seashore Test of Musical Abilities, his performances were at or above the fiftieth percentile on the pitch, loudness, rhythm, and time discrimination subtests. However, his performances in the Timbre and Tonal Memory subtests were at only the fifteenth and twenty-fourth percentile respectively. Sound localization was intact.

His GSR and plethysmogram were monitored to a variety of music. No change in either parameter was seen, not even an "on" response in the skin resistance when the musical stimuli were first presented. After an extensive search, one piece of music was found which successfully eluded the enigmatic process which had deprived him of responsiveness to music. There was a consistent change in resistance while listening to Bach's *Gold-*

berg Variations. This was the only piece of music which he said evoked in him a vestige of his previous emotional responsiveness to music.

This patient therefore did not have epilepsy, much less musicogenic epilepsy but instead had lost his autonomic responses to music.

Narcolepsy

CASE 8. This twenty-eight-year-old graduate student, was referred by her faculty advisor because of short lapses of consciousness in class, and the question was raised if these were episodes of reading epilepsy.

When studied in the Epilepsy Research Laboratory, it became obvious that she had narcolepsy. When reading aloud or while listening to taped lectures in her field of study, she would quickly drowse, fall rapidly into a sound sleep, but could be aroused; if she was not aroused, she awoke spontaneously in five to ten minutes. The EEG showed only sleep activity appropriate to the stage of sleep. Upon questioning, it evolved that when angry or moved to laughter she would have a sensation of weakness of the lower extremities and would try to sit or lie down in these situations. This patient had narcolepsy and cataplexy.

Dyslexia

CASE 9. This unusual referral for possible reading epilepsy, was referred from the Graduate School of the University of Wisconsin. He was a twenty-six-year-old student in his first year of graduate studies. He had attended a small college, where the teaching methodology was heavily pedagogic, and there was no great need for him to read long assignments. The lecture material was sufficient for the examinations. He was in essence told what he would be asked. His faculty advisor in Graduate School was aware of the work being done in the Laboratory and wondered if the patient had reading epilepsy because of his halting reading manner.

The patient had never lost consciousness except for a postural syncope on one occasion. He had had difficulty in reading since the first grade. There was no loss of consciousness or loss of place in following the text. He could read but reported, "it's not easy." He had had eye muscle tonotomy in the past and had been refracted with bifocal glasses with a relatively minor correction.

He was studied in the laboratory to determine whether or not he had reading epilepsy. While reading, he had subjective difficulty, but there were no EEG changes and no evidence, on observing him directly or on reviewing AV tapes, of any disturbance of consciousness or of involuntary movements. He read binocularly, monocularly, vertically, and horizontally using English material, but with frequent errors and particular difficulty with proper names. Digits were read without any difficulty. On the Gettysburg Address, with which he was partially familiar, he proceeded very well in those parts which he recalled, but had difficulty with the reading of particular words like "propriety" (again, however, without evidence of seizures). He was presented with Spanish and found it absolutely impossible to read anything other than the simple, two-letter words such as "la, el." He was presented with patterns of varying types in the laboratory, and these also evoked no EEG changes or clinical seizures.

This young man, therefore, did not have reading epilepsy. His problem was determined by laboratory observations and by the neuropsychological studies to be dyslexic in nature.

Undiagnosed Disturbance of Consciousness

CASE 10. This patient presented the most complicated of the entities confused with reflex epilepsy. Her condition remains undiagnosed, but it certainly is not reading epilepsy. She was a nineteen-year-old female nursing student and was referred with the diagnosis of possible reading epilepsy. She had been well until August, 1969, when she noted spells of blacking out in class. These spells were preceded by a "feeling of being hot all over" and a generalized weakness. She would then stare into space, although she could hear people talking during the spell and remember what they had said. It was felt that these spells could be avoided if someone would shake her. The spells lasted ten to twenty minutes, but the period of actual staring was only two to three minutes. After the spells, she would have generalized tiredness and a mild headache, unresponsive to aspirin, with a sensation of pressure over the head. She denied incontinence or tongue biting during the spells but did note an increase in frequency and severity of the spells during the week preceding her menstrual periods. The attacks were most frequent during classes with lectures and films and where note taking was required. She also noticed that they occurred with greater frequency when deep concentration was required. Spells had occurred while watching television or motion pictures but never while listening to radio or records. The patient stated that after reviewing her old class notes, she believed she had been having these spells since the age of sixteen, as indicated by the breaks in note taking as described below. She had been treated with a variety of medications since the onset of the spells including hydantoin, primidone, amphetamines, dexedrine, Diamox®, and phenobarbital.

Past medical history was negative, as was the family history for any seizure disorder. Physical and neurological examinations and laboratory studies also were normal.

The patient was studied in the Research Laboratory for three weeks, for an average of three and one-half to four hours per day. Her original EEGs were normal. Upon withdrawal of the anticonvulsant medications, however, a dysrhythmia became evident and there were at first some single, low voltage, repetitive, sharp waves, approximately six cycle per second, seen over the right hemisphere, but also infrequently over the left. At times there were phantom spike and wave formations, and sometimes during the special studies, more definitive wave and spike dysrhythmia, especially when the medication had been withheld.

Since her attacks had occurred primarily, although not exclusively, in classrooms, the classroom scene was recreated as closely as possible in the laboratory. For this purpose, medical movies and taped lectures in neurology were played over the speaker system while the patient (a student nurse) took careful notes just as if she had been in class. Thirty-five of her episodes were studied. The onset of these was not clinically clear cut. She

stopped writing, stared ahead, and her face became expressionless, with decreased eye blinks. These episodes lasted from three
to five minutes. During this time she stopped writing completely
or occasionally wrote one word from the lecture, out of context;
for example, an adjective with no following noun. On a few
occasions her pen dribbled on the paper and it was quite easy
to identify by means of the handwriting the point in her notes
where these episodes occurred.

There were no significant EEG changes in these episodes. On
only two of the thirty-five occasions did dysrhythmia occur in
any relationship to the episode. On one occasion, the dysrhythmia
occurred in the middle of the episode and lasted only a second.
On another occasion, it occurred at the very end of a long
episode. It was felt that these were fortuitous occurrences of
spontaneous dysrhythmia during these two episodes. Therefore,
it was not possible to relate this young lady's episodes or attacks
to an EEG dysrhythmia.

Attempts were made to determine if any autonomic responses
were associated with these episodes. Polygraph recording showed
no significant autonomic changes in heart rate, respiratory rate,
GSR, or plethysmographic tracings. When recording during the
two episodes in which the epileptogeniclike dysrhythmia occurred, no accompanying autonomic variables were noted.

There was no significant increase in the number of episodes
when the medication was withdrawn and the classroom situation
repeated. In other words, obtaining an attack in the laboratory
was no more difficult when the patient was taking medication
than when she was off medication. Dexedrine® was given, but
it had no effect. These certainly were not narcoleptic episodes,
and there was no spindling of the EEG during the episodes, but
it was thought that perhaps the amphetamine effects on the
activating system might be of help. However, 15 mg of Dexedrine did not abort the appearance of these spells.

In conclusion, this young lady had an abnormal dysrhythmic
type of EEG record, but it was not possible with careful recording over prolonged periods of time to establish any relationship
between the dysrhythmia and the clinical episodes. The clinical
episodes have not responded to anticonvulsant medication. The

question was raised as to whether they could be functional, but there were certainly no secondary gains involved and her MMPI was normal. She was also seen in psychiatric consultation, and no untoward emotional conflicts were identified. She was studied by projective personality techniques and again was found to be normal.

In summary, this chapter presents some of the problems of the differential diagnosis of reflex epilepsy, and includes entities ranging from anxiety neuroses of various forms to definite organic diseases. The anxiety neuroses may complicate the picture in any of the forms of reflex epilepsy. Recounted here are examples of these resembling the groups of photosensitive, pattern, and musicogenc epilepsy. They could occur as well in others, and a patient with presumed somatosensory-evoked epilepsy presented at the American Neurological Association in 1946 was classified from the movie demonstration as obviously hysterical.

Prolonged observations with standardized testing procedures and careful documentation, especially with audiovisual recording for playback study, are invaluable for resolving these complex problems. The introduction of other techniques, such as the recording of autonomic variables in Cases 6 and 9 also proved highly profitable for research purposes.

CHAPTER 12

BEHAVIORAL THERAPY OF REFLEX EPILEPSY: METHODS AND PRINCIPLES OF APPLICATION

Reflex epilepsy is essentially the predictable occurrence, upon presentation of the appropriate stimulus, of a specific form of clinical seizure, usually with a definitive electroencephalographic concomitant. It is quite logical to assume, therefore, that behavioral methods such as alterations of the presented stimuli could modify and ameliorate the clinical and EEG response, thus leading to a successful behavioral therapy.

The possibility has been raised by others,[1,2,3] as well as by the author, that reflex epilepsy could be a manifestation of a naturally occurring conditional reflex. It was this premise that launched the present series of studies. Because of the early theoretical assumption, the first laboratory attempts at therapy were considered manifestations of extinction of a conditional reflex, hence the use of the term *extinction* in early papers. However, as shown in Chapter 16, reflex epilepsy is not a conditional reflex.

It became apparent as the studies evolved that these naturally occurring reflexes were amenable to behavioral forms of therapy. A review of laboratory data led to the establishment of guidelines and rules for therapy.[4]

Other authors have also described behavioral or conditioning effects in both experimental animal and human epilepsy. The effect of afferent stimuli and arousal upon seizure discharges in humans has been well documented.[5,6,7] Prince[8] has demonstrated this in carefully designed experiments in cats with penicillin-induced epileptogenic foci. Chocholova[9] has shown the effect of adaptation on experimental reflex epilepsy employing rodents with audiogenic seizures.

Efron[10] showed that by a conditioning process it was possible to alter the clinical course in a patient with uncinate seizures. More recently, Sterman and his colleagues[11, 12] have demonstrated the ability of epileptic patients, using biofeedback techniques, to control the electrical activity from the sensory motor cortex.

The single unit studies carried out by the Seattle group[13] demonstrate that in the experimental animal, the epileptic neurons can have their abnormal activity modified by an operant type of conditioning, thus lending further credence to the possible therapeutic effects obtained by behavioral methods in patients.

The studies cited from the literature, both experimental and clinical, show that environmental or behavioral alterations can affect the course of epileptogenic discharges. The University of Wisconsin studies present a systematic therapeutic approach to a carefully studied series of patients with reflex epilepsy.

In the discussion of the classification of reflex epilepsy (Chapter 10) obvious and significant differences were delineated between the simple and the complex types. Basically these differences provide the foundation for many of the following treatment methods. Table XIII presents the methods of therapy employed.

TABLE XIII

BEHAVIORAL THERAPY OF REFLEX EPILEPSY

Methods of Therapy
1. Avoidance of evoking stimuli
   a. Complete
   b. Partial
2. Stimulus alteration: Repeated presentation of altered stimulus
   a. Unilateral presentations
   b. With altered intensity
   c. With or without startle component
   d. With other alterations
3. Threshold alteration: Repeated stimulations in postictal refractory state
4. Vigilance inhibition
5. Avoidance conditioning

METHODS OF CONDITIONING OR BEHAVIORAL THERAPY

Avoidance of the Stimulus

When the individual patient has been carefully studied, and the type of stimulus which evoked his/her seizures determined, it is obvious that the most effective way to treat the patient would be the avoidance or prevention of the occurrence of that stimulus. However, from a practical standpoint, this is usually impossible. Certain exceptions occur, as are described for the specific forms of reflex epilepsy later in this chapter.

Sometimes the avoidance of stimulus on a partial basis may also be effective.

Stimulus Alteration: Repeated Presentation of the Altered Stimulus

This technique involves the repeated presentation of the evoking stimulus altered so that it has lost its epileptogenicity. This alteration can be accomplished by diminishing the intensity of the stimulus so that it is too weak to evoke a seizure or dysrhythmia. In most of the cases of simple reflex epilepsy, the unilateral presentation of the evoking stimulus does not induce a seizure or dysrhythmia. The stimulus therefore can be repeatedly given unilaterally as a method of alteration. In those patients in whom a startle component is necessary for the seizure evocation, the patient can be apprized of the delivery of the stimulus, thus initially removing the startle component. Under these conditions, the stimulus fails to evoke dysrhythmia or seizures. Other alterations are possible as noted in the particular forms of reflex epilepsy.

Threshold Alteration: Repeated Stimulations in the Postictal Refractory State

In certain patients with reflex epilepsy, particularly when the seizures are temporal lobe or major motor in type, postictal refractory phases are observed. This postictal refractory phase can be employed for behavioral or conditioning treatment. The patient is exposed to the evoking stimulus and the seizure (usually temporal lobe in type) is induced; the stimulus is continuously repeated during the seizure, during the postictal refractory period, and until clinical and electroencephalographic normality have returned. This method employs the higher seizure threshold which occurs in the postictal state. As the threshold gradually approaches its usual level, the presentations are continued.

When the evoked seizures are minor and the refractory phase persists for an extended period of time, the refractory phase can also be employed as a therapeutic measure. The patient can self-induce his seizures under controlled situations and continue his daily routine being certain he will not have another inadvertently evoked seizure.

Vigilance Inhibition

When the previously described methods of behavioral therapy are unavailable or unsuccessful, and when the patient is in control of the stimulus presentation as in reading epilepsy, it is possible to use a vigilance inhibition technique. This consists of the signaling of the occurrence of events related to the seizure evoking process and blocks to some extent the occurrence of the seizures.

Avoidance Conditioning

In patients who self-induce their seizures, it is possible, by the administration of skin shocks, to teach the patient to avoid the evoking stimulus. This method is of limited value, for use in patients who are totally incapable of cooperating with other behavioral techniques and in whom seizure induction is so frequent as to be almost continuous. This method can be employed to break through the patient's self-inducing activity in order to study his total intellectual and other assets.

APPLICATION OF THE BEHAVIORAL METHODS OF TREATMENT TO THE VARIOUS FORMS OF REFLEX EPILEPSY

The various methods of behavioral treatment cannot be applied indiscriminately to each and every form of reflex epilepsy. Also, the application of the methods vary in the different forms of reflex epilepsy. These variations are dependent upon the nature of the evoking stimulus, whether the reflex epilepsy is simple or complex, and whether the stimulus presentation is under the control of the patient. The application of the behavioral treatment is now considered in relation to each form of reflex epilepsy.

Visually Induced Epilepsy

Of the methods of treatment, three cannot be applied. These are avoidance of stimulus, threshold alteration, and vigilance inhibition. The difficulties which prevent the use of these methods are detailed.

Avoidance of the stimulus is not a practical way in which to treat these patients. It is impossible for the patient to avoid flickering light, distinct patterns, eye closure, or the presentation of a particular color in the environment and still lead a normal existence.

Employment of the postictal refractory phase or *threshold alteration* is also not a feasible way for treating patients with photosensitivity, pattern, or eye closure seizures. The seizures evoked in the laboratory are almost invariably minor seizures of the petit mal type. If the stroboscopic stimulation is continued, the seizures will recur (*see* Fig. 53). In this study there was not the opportunity to employ continung stimulations in patients with major motor seizures evoked by photic stimulation, and it was not considered justifiable to pursue the photic stimulation to the point of inducing a major motor seizure in order to test this possibility. However, if during the laboratory study a patient should have a major seizure upon the presentation of photic stimulation, that point could be clarified by continuing the photic stimulation through the postical state.

Vigilance therapy has no role in the treatment of the visually induced seizures. Vigilance is obviously impossible since the patient cannot predict the occurrence of the stimulus and thus put into action the vigilance technique. Moreover, administering auditory clicks simultaneously with the stroboscopic stimulations prior to conditioning in no way inhibits the development of dysrhythmia or seizures (see Chapter 13).

Stimulus alteration is the most effective method for behavioral treatment in visually induced epilepsies. This consists of the repeated presentation of the altered evoking stimulus. Since monocular or unilateral presentations do not evoke seizures in most of the patients with photosensitivity, pattern, or eye-closure induced dysrhythmia, this technique can be used in the behavioral treatment.[14] Repeated presentations do not evoke the dysrhythmia and after these repeated monocular presentations, bilateral stimulations also do not evoke seizures (Fig. 54). This method can only be used in patients who are monocularly insensitive, have had relatively few or no major seizures, have a relatively small range of photosensitivity, and have in addition, no other forms of visually induced epilepsy.

A high degee of cooperation is necessary. The patients must maintain a soft velvet patch, carefully positioned over one eye so as not to permit a light leak. As noted before, if they allow the patch to slip and thus obtain some binocular stimulations, they become monocularly sensitive. Therefore, determination of

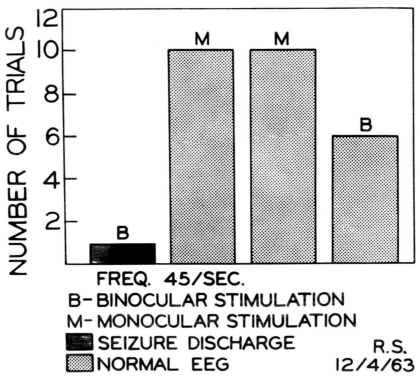

Figure 54. Repeated monocular stimulations for behavioral treatment of photosensitivity. Binocular stimulations evoked seizure discharges. After ten presentations of monocular stimulation to each eye (total twenty trials) binocular stimulations did not evoke seizures. Case 2, Chapter 2. Reprinted from *Arch Neurol, 11*:603, 1964.

the ability of the patient to cooperate is an important factor in selecting this mode of therapy.

The stimulations are administered in the laboratory with EEG monitoring and are given for fifteen-minute periods, first to one eye and then to the other, alternated in this way daily for two morning and afternoon sessions each lasting one and one-half to two hours. Between sessions, the patients wear an eye patch over one eye until after the fourth or fifth session when a test is made by binocular stimulations. These usually do not evoke a dysrhythmia after this period of time, and the patients are then in the intervening period, allowed to go, without wearing the patch. During this process it is of critical importance that the patients realize the necessity of not moving the patch from one eye to the other until the stroboscope has been turned off. The entire process usually requires about two weeks.

However, for most patients with photosensitivity, the technique chosen was that of altering the intensity of the stimulus.[15, 16] Patients with monocular sensitivity, with more frequent or severe seizures, with wide ranges of frequencies evoking their seizures, or with concomitant pattern epilepsy are best treated by this method of stimulus alteration.

The technique which was devised for this is the differential light intensity method. This consists of the use, for the therapeutic process, of the reciprocal relationship between ambient room light and stroboscopic intensity (Figs. 55, 56). The ambient light was increased to the point where the stroboscopic flashes were barely perceptible. This was accomplished by placing the stroboscope behind an opaque glass, flanked on either side by photofloods, with a rheostatic control supplying the power to the photofloods. At the maximum intensity of light from the photofloods, a light level of 600 footcandles was obtained at the bridge of the patient's nose. Gradually diminishing the current to the photofloods allowed the stroboscope to become more and more apparent. In this entire process, the patient and his/her EEGs were monitored by AV tape recording. The AV monitor is especially useful for the operator, for he can visualize both patient and EEG quickly for his decision making.

Originally, the stroboscope and ambient light control were

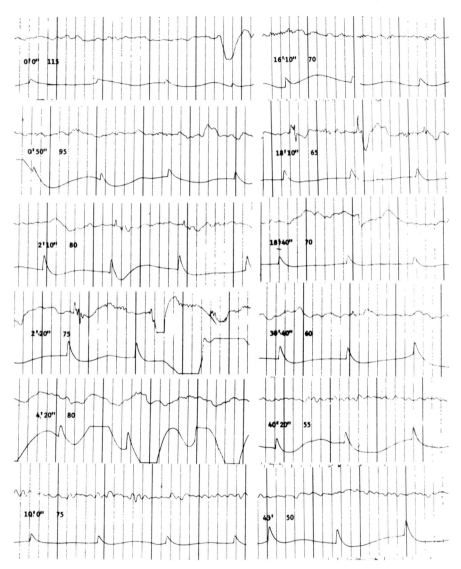

Figure 55. Differential light intensity method of behavioral treatment of photosensitivity. Time duration is indicated by numbers beginning 0'00". Other numbers indicate settings on rheostat controlling ambient room light. At 115, ambient light is 600 footcandles and at 50 is about 30 foot candles. Upper tracings are EEGs. Lower tracing is photoelectric cell pickup to indicate administration of single light flash stimulations. Case 3, Chapter 2.

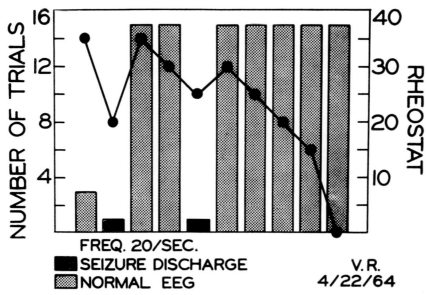

Figure 56. Effect of repeated presentation of evoking photic stimulus with differential light intensity. Rheostat values indicate ambient room light. 40 is equivalent to 200 footcandles. Binocular presentations evoke no dysrhythmia. At lower levels, dysrhythmias occur. With careful decrease of ambient light and monitoring for occurrence of dysrhythmia, it is possible to reduce ambient light to 0. Reprinted from *Arch Neurol, 11*:603, 1964.

operated manually and the operator had to make the decision to alter the stimulus upon the appearance of the significant dysrhythmia evoked by the photic stimulation. Obviously, this technique was fatiguing and difficult in that it required rapid decisions to be made as to whether or not the display of the EEG was a dysrhythmia or a movement artifact (which frequently occurred in such prolonged periods of therapy). If dysrhythmias were evoked by photic stimulation, it was necessary to cease the stimulation almost within the reaction time limitations of the investigator in order to avoid a clinical seizure. The fact that the process required two to two and one-half hours twice a day over a period of two weeks to accomplish made the fatigue factor unbearable.

For these reasons, a biofeedback mechanism was devised, and the entire process was computer automated. This was accomplished at first in a pilot program by sending the EEG transmission across the University of Wisconsin campus to the Cybernetics Laboratory of Doctor K. U. Smith by way of a leased telephone line. By way of return telephone line, the computer controlled the ambient light source and stroboscope. This was proved feasible, and later, a special computer was built for this process and placed in the laboratory (Fig. 57A). This operated a unit containing a stroboscope flanked by photofloods (Fig. 57B).*

This computer monitors and writes out the EEG and at the same time writes out and controls the step intervals in room light and stroboscopic stimulation (Fig. 58). The frequency of the stroboscopic stimulations is preset, and the computer is assigned the control of the stroboscope on-off switch and of rheostatic control for the ambient light. The sensitivity of the computer usually is set to register spiking discharges for time within two hundred milliseconds and for amplitude. In the course of the conditioning process if, as the ambient light is decreased, a dysrhythmia occurs, the computer immediately stops the stroboscope, resets the ambient light levels several steps higher and begins the entire process again (Fig. 59).

Sometimes a "hang-up" occurs, and the computer automation fails to pass a particular point of lower light intensity. Since the stimulations are given binocularly and since most patients do not have a dysrhythmia evoked by monocular stimulation, patching of one eye can be employed for three to five runs through these steps of light intensity and a return then made to binocular stimulations.

Whether the eyes are open or closed is also important. Some patients are not sensitive in one of these two conditions, or are much more sensitive with eyes closed than open or vice versa. In these situations it is important that no change be made in the lower steps of light intensity from a less noxious to a more noxious situation. For example, when a patient who is more sensitive with eyes closed is being treated with eyes open and

---

* These units were manufactured by Instrument and Controls System, Incorporated, 129 Laura Drive, Addison, Illinois.

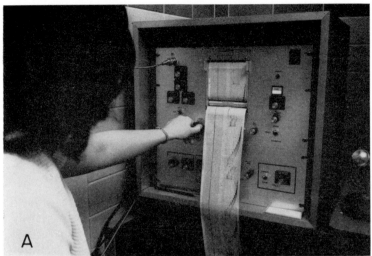

Figure 57A. Computer automation and other equipment in control room. Technician operating equipment and in position to view patient through two-way window. Technician's hand is on computer automation equipment which is in control of stimulus administration while monitoring patient's EEG. Cathode screen (not shown) also permits visual monitoring by technician of patient's EEG's. These demonstrations more nearly approximate usual EEG demonstrations. This permits technician to make decisions between artifact and abnormal EEG recordings. Note microphone which can be "opened" to allow communication with patient.

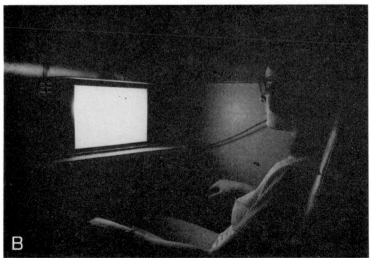

Figure 57B. Patient in cubicle, wearing specially designed glasses and viewing panel with stroboscopic stimulations and ambient room light.

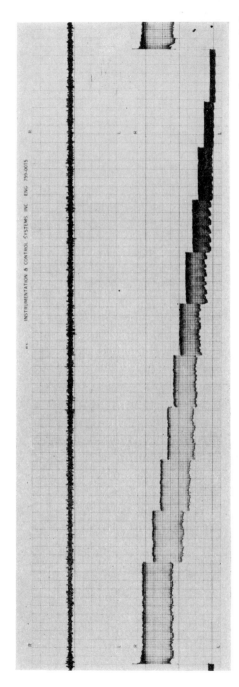

Figure 58. Computer automation print-out of conditioning process. Top line is EEG print-out. Each vertical line represents seconds. Lower line shows, in steps, the decreases from 600 footcandles of ambient light intensity at left to darkness (except for stroboscope) at right. Far right is the beginning or a new cycle. The vertical write-out in second channel represents the stroboscopic frequencies. There is no evoked dysrhythmia, and the steps in conditioning are uneventful.

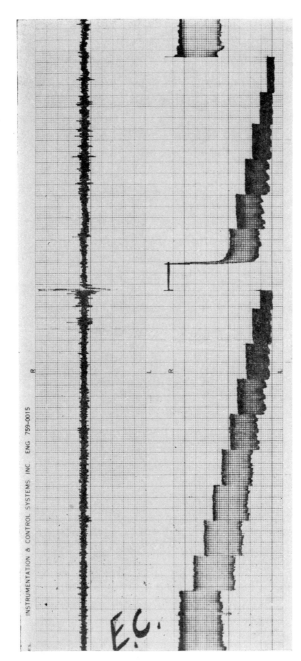

Figure 59. Computer automation print-out of conditioning process. Channels as in Figure 58. Evoked dysrhythmia results in interruption of photic stimulation and resetting of levels of ambient room light several levels higher. Conditioning proceeds uneventually through remainder of steps and a new cycle is then begun. "EC" indicates patient has eyes closed.

the light intensity has been reduced to a few foot candles, if he closes his eyes he is very apt to have a dysrhythmia evoked.

It is better to begin the process with eyes closed, for this is more comfortable for the patient. The procedure is continued until no dysrhythmia is evoked. The process is then repeated with the patient in the eyes-open state.

When a "hang-up" occurs, the state which is less sensitive or which has already been treated can be employed. For example, in the patient who is no longer sensitive to stimuli with eyes closed, when the computer automation fails to get past a particular point with eyes opened, the introduction of several complete therapeutic runs with eyes closed may allow the process to proceed in the eyes-open state. Also, the trials can be started with eyes open and, at the step before that in which the dysrhythmia was evoked, the patient is ordered to close his eyes. The eyes are kept closed during the remainder of that process. After several trials the step process can be carried one increment further each time, with eyes open, until the entire range of 600 foot candles to 0 ambient light is reached (Fig. 60).

In each of the patients, the frequency range of stroboscopic stimulations which evoked seizures was carefully determined. The presentation of the altered stimulus was begun, usually in the center of the range. For example, if a patient's sensitive range was from fifteen to twenty-five flashes per second, the original treatments were begun at twenty flashes per second. When the therapeutic process rendered these stimulations innocuous, a band of roughly eighteen to twenty-two flashes per second had become innocuous. It was necessary then to repeat the treatment process for the remaining frequencies which evoked dysrhythmia.

Treatment could also be begun outside the sensitive frequency range (Fig. 61). One could begin at thirty-eight to forty flashes per second in the patient with a noxious range of fifteen to thirty-five flashes per second. After a series of stimulations, the flash rate could be decreased and the sensitive range approached. The same can be done at the lower limit of the sensitive range. This, however, as can be readily appreciated, increases the treatment time since it makes use of only half of

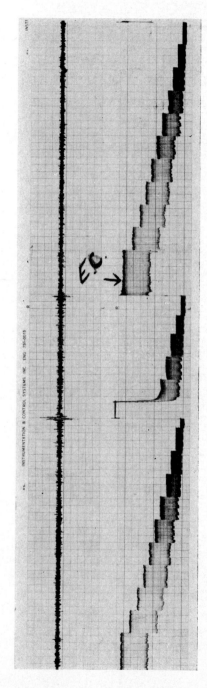

Figure 60. Computer automation print-out of conditioning process. Channels as in Figures 58 and 59. Patient being run with eyes open. After repeated attempts in which stroboscopic stimulations were interrupted because of evoked dysrhythmia, the patient was told to close her eyes (EC) and the process of conditioning could be continued.

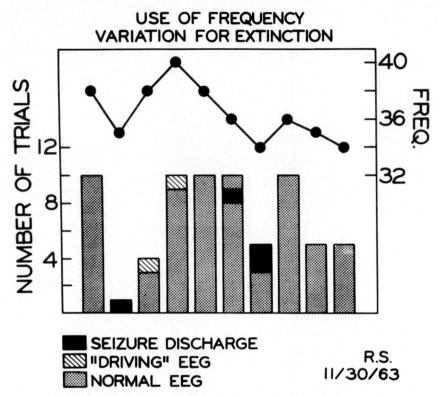

Figure 61. Demonstrates use of frequency variation in treatment process. Patient has dysrhythmia and seizures evoked at 2x 35 per second stimulation. Beginning above that frequency and with repeated stimulations, it is possible to deliver stimulations at 35 per second. This is obviously a more difficult process. Reprinted from *Arch Neurol, 11*:603, 1964.

the slight generalization (about five cycles per second). This technique, however, could be used in a difficult treatment problem.

It has been noted that patients with photosensitivity are less apt to have evoked dysrhythmias while asleep. During these long sessions, patients sometimes fall asleep. These sleep states can also be used in the treatment process, but it is necessary to avoid a sudden waking of the patient, particularly at the lower steps of ambient light. When one wishes to wake the patient, it is best to wait until the ambient light has returned to maximum.

Certain psychological or emotional factors are apparent in the course of these treatment sessions. These include the effect of the particular therapist, the apprehension of the patients if they learn the meaning of the interruption of the decreasing light steps, and a peculiar, transient resistance, almost a "negative transference."

The peculiar resistance usually becomes apparent about the third day. Patients come slowly to the laboratory, complain of being tired, are irritable, and sometimes cry. Some show this phase by being indifferent and going to sleep. The laboratory personnel explain this situation to the patients as a normal occurrence during this prolonged therapy.

The placing of the patient alone in a separate, sound-deadened cubicle is necessary to avoid the first two difficulties just described. If the patient is aware of the presence or absence of the physician, or that only the technician is present, the patient attaches particular significance to this. He/she is often concerned if the responsible physician is not present or, conversely, may interpret his appearance as an indication that all is not going well. Also, the patient senses the most subtle signal between physician and technician regarding the significance of the computer alteration of the ambient light and of the stroboscopic stimulation. It is quite likely that the failure in Case 35 was based on this awareness.

For these reasons, a special room was constructed, placing the patient in a cubicle and all controlling equipment outside the cubicle. Only the stroboscope and the ambient light sources were in the cubicle with the patient (*see* Fig. 57B). Communication was always possible from the patient by intercom and, when desired, from the operator to the patient, by opening a switch. It is also important not to speak or disturb the patient at the more critical parts of the therapeutic stimulation. Unless absolutely necessary, no communication was made from the control room to the cubicle until the ambient light was brought back by computer automation to the maximum.

Pattern dysrhythmia can be treated employing the same computer operation. The pattern is projected onto the opaque glass in front of the stroboscope and photofloods. Thus the pattern also is at first barely perceptible in the bright light and gradually becomes more evident.

Most of the pattern epilepsy patients were also photosensitive, so their therapeutic processes could be combined and treated simultaneously. In treatment of patients with photosensitive seizures only, the conditioning seems to move more smoothly when there is an image on the screen or other distractions present. Travelogues and other similar slides are now projected on the face of the screen, even if the patient is only being treated for photosensitivity.

In pattern epilepsy, changes of focus[17] can also be used in the conditioning process. The pattern can be presented out of focus and gradually brought into focus. If done carefully, this can be accomplished without eliciting a dysrhythmia or seizure.

The pattern presentation with varying focus and light has been standardized in the laboratory. The various patterns have been filmed on Super 8 mm film, beginning at a very low illumination level and in poor focus, and gradually approaching sharp focus and brightness. These films are on cassettes and can be projected on a screen before the patient.

In eye closure dysrhythmia, since monocular patching prevents the occurence of the dysrhythmia, the patients can be treated by repeated blinking with one eye patched.[17] Since eye closure dysrhythmia does not occur in the dark, the patient can be instructed to blink repeatedly in a very dim light. The differential light intensity technique is thus reversed, beginning with darkness and proceeding to the 600 foot candles of ambient light.

Avoidance conditioning was employed in the laboratory only in the patient with seizures evoked by looking at the color red or at his hand (Case 39). Since this was a complex type of visually induced epilepsy, there was a strong suggestion that threshold alteration was in evidence. It was noted that the patient's first seizure in the morning, usually when hunching over a red object rather than his hand, was a tonic seizure lasting about ten seconds. The continued hunching over the red object would evoke myoclonic jerks which gradually diminished in severity until he was no longer able to evoke a seizure. He would then wander about the laboratory for five to ten minutes until he could repeat the process.

This strongly suggested that threshold alteration could have been employed in therapy. However, because of his retardation and hyperactivity it was not possible to carry such therapy out in the necessary systematic fashion. Since the patient's purposeful, "goal interested" activities revolved exclusively on seizure-induction phenomena, and since there was a question as to whether if he were not so employed he might be trainable or educable to some degree, the avoidance conditioning was used.

By using a remote control device with a shock box attached to his thigh for a period of three days, he was conditioned not to stare at red objects or at his hand in order to induce seizures. He could pick up red objects as well as objects of any other color and play with them, but if he attempted to hunch over them to induce a seizure, he was administered a shock. After about five hours in the laboratory and six avoidance shocks, he gave up hunching over red objects and played with these as well as others for the first time in years. He then began hunching over his hand in order to induce seizures. Again the same technique was used. Skin shocks were administered whenever he hunched over his hand to evoke a seizure. This dissuaded him from the self-induction of seizures. He was then studied in depth at the Wisconsin Central Colony and Training School with the hope that he might be found educable or trainable. However, after six weeks at the Colony, it was determined that the child was not trainable, much less educable. His family preferred to have him enjoy his only "purposeful" behavior, that is, the induction of minor seizures.

Auditory-Evoked Epilepsy: Simple Type

In the simple type of auditory-evoked epilepsy (for example, acousticomotor startle epilepsy), *avoidance of the evoking stimulus* is impossible. These stimuli arise from the environment and are unpredictable. The backfiring of an engine, the sudden blowing of a car horn, or the slamming of a door are examples of the kind of evoking stimuli which cannot be predicted or avoided. It would be necessary to place the patient into a soundproof or sound-deadened environment in order to avoid the stimuli. This is, of course, impractical.

The method of *stimulus alteration* is the one of choice in the simple type of auditory-evoked epilepsy. It can be accomplished by administering the stimuli monaurally through earphones much as in the monocular treatment of photosensitivity (Figs. 62, 63). The unilateral sensory stimulation is given repeatedly over periods of one and one-half to two hours in two sessions per day, and samplings of binaural stimulations are then tested after four or five sessions (Fig. 64). As noted before, it is

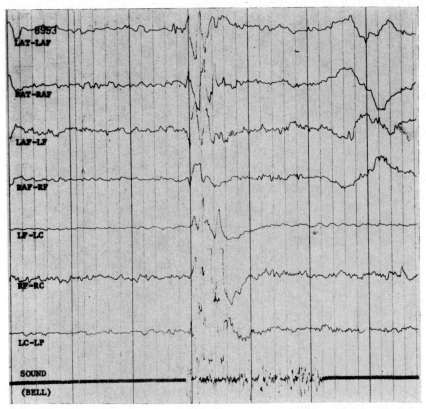

Figure 62.   Acousticomotor epilepsy. Myoclonic seizure evoked by sudden binaural startling presentation of sound of bell. Lower channel is sound indicator. Changes in EEG channel are artifactual as demonstrated by Anectine studies. Patient had generalized myoclonic seizure. Reprinted from *Neurology* © 1965 by The New York Times Media Company, Inc.

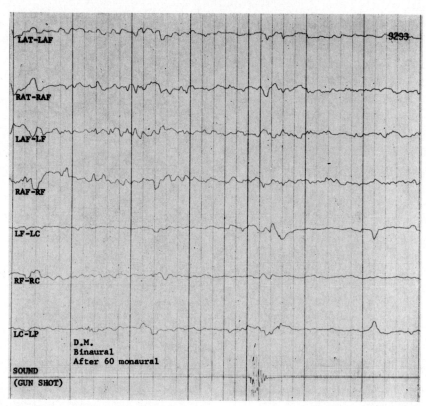

Figure 63. Same patient. Monaural presentation of sudden startling sound. No clinical response.

important that the monaural presentations not exceed a level of 60 decibels, for at and above this level there is bone conduction to the opposite ear. Thus the stimuli are in fact binaural even though technically administered to only one ear.

Stimulus alteration can also be accomplished by altering the intensity of the stimulus. This can be done by presentation either through earphones or in the free fields while maintaining the sound levels below that intensity which had been previously determined necessary to evoke the dysrhythmia or seizure. These altered stimuli are presented repeatedly and gradually increased in intensity. Thus it is possible to surpass the previously determined threshold for evocation of dysrhythmias and seizures.

The stimuli are administered in free fields by playing prepared

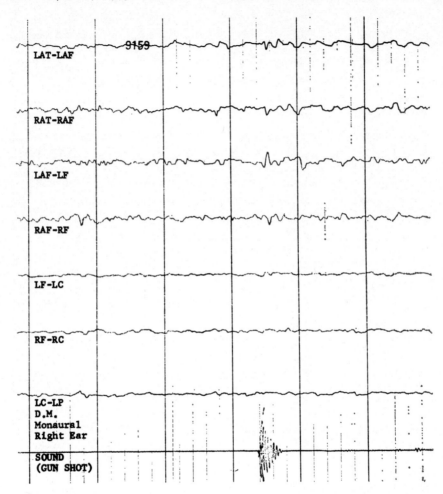

Figure 64. Same patient. Binaural presentation of same sound, same sound level. After sixty monaural presentations. No clinical seizure evoked. Reprinted from *Neurology* © 1965 by The New York Times Media Company, Inc.

audiotapes over a stereo tape recorder and using speakers balanced for the position of the patient in the laboratory. The prepared tapes have the sounds randomized in time and with sounds of gradually increasing intensity. In the early studies, only a single sound in a series, was presented, for example, a particular bell, rifle shot, sound of a dropped metal dish, or sonic boom. This particular sound was presented until it no longer evoked dysrhythmia or seizures, even though the sound level had surpassed by far the original threshold. After the initial presentation was completed, another sound was introduced in the same way. The procedure was repeated until all known evoking sounds had been included in the therapeutic process. In later studies, included in randomized form at the beginning of treatment were all known or suspected sounds. This simplified the treatment process.

The component of startle is necessary for the evocation of many of the simple forms of auditory-induced epilepsy. The elimination of the role of startle also serves as a method of altering the stimulus presentation. The method is explained to the patient, and the tape recorder used to present the sound stimuli is placed in front of the patient so that he can see it in operation. The patient is well aware that stimuli will be presented. When the therapeutic process is well underway, unexpected stimuli are used to test the efficacy of the conditioning. For example, in the laboratory is a loud electric alarm type bell. This can be activated by a remote switch and is one of the devices used to sample the efficacy of the therapeutic process. The use of the bell of course introduces a startle element.

Regardless of the method of alteration of stimulus, *the principle is the same, consisting of repeated presentations of the altered stimulus followed by the introduction of the unaltered stimulus.*

The monaural or unilateral presentation method is unnatural and therefore not the ideal primary method of treatment. Working in free fields is far more preferable and natural. The combination of the free field method with the elimination of the startle factor is the best method of treatment for the simple types of auditory-evoked seizures. The monaural presentations, however, can be employed if necessary to overcome difficulties in the treatment process, in much the same manner as monocular presentations are used during the differential light intensity technique in photosensitivity when the treatment process is not progressing saisfactorily.

The *vigilance inhibition* method of therapy is not available for the treatment of this type of epilepsy. The patient would have to be aware of the impending presentation of the stimulus in order to employ vigilance. This of course is impossible in view of the startle nature of the stimulus presentation.

The *threshold alteration* method cannot be employed in this type of epilepsy. Neither the minor seizures of startle epilepsy nor the tonic seizures evoked by sound are followed by a post-ictal refractory phase. Repeated presentations are ineffective; for example, in the tonic seizures evoked by sound, repeated presentations of the stimuli aggravate the involuntary movements.

Avoidance conditioning is not applicable for these patients since they are not self-inducing their seizures.

Auditory-Evoked Epilepsy: Complex Type

In the complex types of auditory-evoked reflex epilepsy, only the threshold alteration method can be employed at the present time.

Avoidance of stimulus is impossible when the stimuli consist of telephone transmissions or voice characteristics. The latter patient would have had to remain at home, conversing only with her husband and a few people whose voices she knew would not evoke seizures. She would have had to avoid church, stores, social events, and, indeed, any communication with unknown persons.

Stimulus alteration is likewise not feasible since the exact parameters of the stimuli which evoked the dysrhythmias or seizures in these patients could not be determined.

Vigilance inhibition therapy also cannot be employed in these forms of reflex epilepsy since the patients are not in control of the stimulus presentation.

Avoidance conditioning could serve no purpose since these patients were not self-inducing their attacks and had no secondary gain from the seizures.

Threshold alteration is therefore the behavioral treatment of choice for the patients with the complex type of auditory-evoked reflex epilepsy. This technique includes the evocation of seizures and the use of the postictal refractory phase,[19] as demonstrated by the laboratory studies in the patient with voice-induced epilepsy (Case 10,Chapter 3). This patient had seizures evoked by the voices of three specific radio announcers. While other voices also evoked seizures, these were difficult to identify, as she frequently had seizures in public places when many people were speaking. However, the relationship of seizures to the voices of these three specific radio announcers was unquestionable and was confirmed in the laboratory. Table XIV shows the effect of the presentations of the voice stimuli of these announcers. When the presentations of the first voice no longer induced seizures, the second voice stimulus was presented. After the second voice failed to evoke seizures, the third voice stimulus was presented.

The failure of the initial presentation of the first voice to evoke a seizure is an example of the varying stimulus response time in the complex type of reflex epilepsy. On the second presentation, a typical seizure was evoked. However, following this, the evoked seizures became progressively less severe. There were some EEG dysrhythmias evoked, but after two hours neither seizures nor dysrhythmia were evoked by the presentation of this particular voice. The second and third voices evoked much less dramatic clinical and EEG responses than did those of the first voice. This indicates some generalization of the effect of the conditioning for the first voice.

Musicogenic Epilepsy

In modern society, the *avoidance of this stimulus* is virtually impossible. The introduction of battery-operated transistor radios and the widespread use of music in various places of business and professional enterprises presents an almost constant stimulation by music. There is, nonetheless, a report of a patient who scrupulously avoided music for five years and then was again able to listen to music.[20] However, the inability to avoid exposure to music becomes a severe handicap for the patient with musicogenic epilepsy, and two of the study patients lost their employment because of seizures inadvertently evoked by music.

Vigilance inhibition plays no role in the prevention of seizures. Various methods of distraction used by the patients when listening to particular noxious numbers did not prevent the occurrence of seizures. This is not surprising in view of the fact that

TABLE XIV

TREATMENT OF VOICE-INDUCED EPILEPSY

Rx. Sessions			Location	C.S. Presented	No. of Presentations	Clinical Response	EEG Response
- 27-67	Time		Cond. Lab.	R.Z. tape 1	1	0	N
am			Cond. Lab.	R.Z. tape 1	2	Focal Sx	L.T. Dys.
			Cond. Lab.	R.Z. tape 1	3	3 slight focal sx.	3 L.T. Dys.
			Cond. Lab.	R.Z. tape 1	4	1 very slight sx.	3 L.T. Dys.
			Cond. Lab.	R.Z. tape 1	5	1 very slight sx	2 L.T. Dys.
	2^0		Cond. Lab.	R.Z. tape 1	6-9	0	N
pm	1^020		Cond. Lab.	R.Z. tape 1	1-5	0	N
	1^0		Pt's Rm.	R.Z. tape 1	1&2	0	——
11-28-67	2^0		Cond. Lab.	R.Z. tape 1	1-6	0	N
	1^0		Pt's Rm.	R.Z. tape 1	1-4	0	——
11-29-67	2^0		Cond. Lab.	R.Z. tape 1	1	0	N
am			Cond. Lab.	R.Z. tape 2	1-3	0	N
			Cond. Lab.	E.D. tape	1	Focal sx slight	L.T. Dys.
				E.D. tape	2	0	N
				E.D. tape	3	Focal sx slight	L.T. Dys.
	2^030			E.D. tape	4	0	N
pm			Cond. Lab.	R.H.	1	Aura	N
			Cond. Lab.	R.H.	2	0	N
	3^0		Cond. Lab.	R.Z., E.D., & R.H.	1	0	N
	3^0		Pt's Rm.	R.Z., E.D., & R.H.	3	0	——

Total Time—Lab. 15^025
TotalTime   Pt's Rm. 5^0

From Forster, F. M., Hansotia, P., Cleeland, C. S., and Ludwig, A.: A case of voice-induced epilepsy treated by conditioning. *Neurology, 19*:325, 1969.

seizures can be evoked when the patients hear music during sleep. Also, an awareness of the music on the part of the patient, even when awake, is not necessary for seizure evocation.

Avoidance conditioning obviously could play no role in the treatment of this condition since the patient is not in control of the stimulus presentation.

The *alteration of stimulus* technique can be employed, but it

TABLE XV

STIMULUS ALTERATION BY MIXTURES OF SIMPLIFIED AND ORCHESTRA MUSIC

	Simplified (Organ)	Complete Version (Orchestra)	Time	Days	EEG	Clinical
Conditioning	100%	——	14-¼⁰	5	0	0
Conditioning	66⅔-100%	0-33⅓%	4-½⁰	3	0	0
Test Trial	50%	50%	7"	—	+	+
Conditioning	66⅔-100%	0-33⅓%	10-¼⁰	3	0	0
Test Trial	50%	50%	5' (X3)	—	0	0
Conditioning	50-100%	0-50%	10⁰	6	0	0
Test Trial	33⅓%	66⅔%	5'	—	0	0
Conditioning	33⅓-100%	0-66⅔%	10⁰	3	0	0
Test Trial	0	100%	5'	—	0	0
Conditioning	0	100%	used as innocuous music thereafter			

is not the method of choice.[21] The alteration technique was demonstrated in the first study patient with musicogenic epilepsy. He had seizures to a kind of music popular in the 1930s. After prolonged playing of widely divergent musical types which did not evoke seizures or dysrhythmia, a seizure occurred when a particular evoking number was played.

But when the patient listened to this particular number as rendered in simplified form by an electric organ or computer, no seizure was evoked. After repeated presentations of this simplified rendition, the orchestrated rendition continued to evoke seizures. The simplified form was again employed, and, after repeated playing, the orchestrated version was introduced, at first in a ratio of two bars to every ninety-eight of the organ music. The precentage of exposure was gradually increased. Table XV shows the manner in which this was accomplished. After fifty hours of listening, it was possible for the patient to listen to the entire orchestrated version without having a seizure. As noted in Table XV, at one point, the treatment proceeded too rapidly; a seizure was evoked, and, of necessity, the treatment was then continued at a slower pace.

The patient had no seizures when he heard orchestrations sufficiently similar to that particular version to permit some generalization. However, other renditions, including vocal numbers, evoked seizures. Using similar laborious techniques, it was possible to produce a conditioned effect by introducing other elements and components; male voices, female voices, and combined male and female voices.

Nevertheless, the syncopated version of the original number still evoked seizures. He was presented with both the syncopated and standard version played simultaneously, beginning with the standard version played so loudly that the syncopated version could barely be heard. The intensity of the syncopated version was gradually increased while the sound intensity of the standard version was decreased. After fifteen presentations with these gradual changes, he was able to listen to the syncopated version alone without seizure evocation.

This study showed that stimulus alteration could be employed in at least some instances of musicogenic epilepsy, but it is obviously too time consuming. It should be noted that stimulus alteration would be the treatment of choice in patients whose seizures are evoked by a particular note or chord. These cases would be of the simple type of musicogenic epilepsy. To date the author and his colleagues have not seen such a patient.

Szobor and Frater[22] reported a case of musicogenic epilepsy who was permitted to listen to the radio each day, beginning with short periods of time and gradually increasing the amounts until he was able to listen for as long as he wished. This is probably an example of stimulus alteration by changing the duration of presentation. The efficacy of such a procedure depends upon two factors: first, that the patient's seizures do not occur too soon after the beginning presentation of the music, and second and most important, that the continuing increments be of the appropriate type of music, i.e. the kind of music responsible for the patient's seizures. In the United States of America, this would be difficult because of the wide variety of types of music presented by the media.

In the treatment of musicogenic epilepsy, no further attempt was made in the laboratory to engage in the stimulus alteration technique for two reasons: (a) the process is too time consuming, and (b) a more rapidly effective method of treatment was found.

The *threshold alteration method* is the behavioral treatment of choice in the complex type of musicogenic epilepsy.[23] The scanning tapes described in Chapter 4 are presented to patients suspected of musicogenic epilepsy. These tapes are continued until a seizure occurs. During the seizure, during the postictal confused period, and during the gradual return to normality of both the clinical state of the patient and the EEG, the same musical number is continued. It is continuously played, usually for about one hour. A second seizure has never occurred in the laboratory during this period of time.

After completion of the conditioning process for that particular musical number, testing continues, using the remainder of the scanning tapes. Explorations are also made into types of music similar to that which evoked the seizure. For example, if a patient's seizures are evoked by the ballets of Tschiakovsky, his symphonies are presented as well as ballets by other composers. When another musical number is encountered which evokes either seizures or dysrhythmia, the therapeutic process of repeated presentations is again instituted.

Occasionally, the presentation of a music number may evoke dysrhythmias which do not proceed into a complete electrical and clinical seizure. The repeated presentations, in sequence, of that number will lead to a gradual decrease in the number of evoked spiking dysrhythmias. Not only will the quantity of the dysrhythmias decrease but also the quality. The spiking dysrhythmia becomes less and less sharp, and after repeated presentations, usually ten to fifteen, is no longer evident. This method is just as efficacious as is the method of repeated presentations during and after an evoked seizure.

It is important to study the effects of many types of music. Evoking stimuli may also be found in music quite different from that which is the obvious or primary offender. It is also necessary to include seasonal music (for example Christmas and patriotic music) as well as the kind of religious music appropriate for the patient.

An attempt was usually made to limit the therapeutic sessions to two weeks in order to minimize the fatigue factor for both patient and investigator. For special music, such as Christmas music, an appropriate session would be rescheduled prior to the advent of this type of music in stores and over the radio.

Reading Epilepsy

It is possible to employ the method of *avoidance of stimulus* in reading epilepsy, since the patient is in control of the administration of the stimulus. Casual reading of a few words as a newspaper headline, a sign board, or the title of a book is not a sufficient stimulus to evoke seizures. The patient must be consciously reading for a period of time. Therefore, the patient could, by avoidance of the stimulus, prevent the occurrence of seizures. In general, however, this is too high a price to pay for the control of seizures.

Nevertheless, the study included two patients who have applied this method. Brief resumes of these cases follow:

CASE 1. This thirty-three-year-old Sioux Indian male was diagnosed as having reading epilepsy in 1958. He had two seizures while serving in the United States Navy. The first episode occurred while he was reading a book. He noted involuntary jerking of his tongue and shoulder but continued to read and became unconscious. He was taken to the Naval hospital where he awoke, disoriented and tired. One week later, again while he was reading, he was found by a colleague, slumped forward and with shaking of all extremities. He was taken to the hospital and on awaking was tired and disoriented. He had been studied in two Naval hospitals, including Great Lakes, and discharged from the Navy with the diagnosis of reading epilepsy.

From 1958 to 1964, he severely limited his reading. Occasionally when he did become involved in reading, he noticed some tongue jerking and would immediately stop, thus preventing the progress into a major seizure. Since 1964, he had not read anything more than headlines or street signs. During this time he was working as an electrician for the Bureau of Indian Affairs and was taking no anticonvulsant medication. Because the possibility of promotion would entail reading manuals, he sought advice as to whether or not his reading epilepsy was still present.

His family history, past history, physical and neurological examinations were all normal.

He was presented in 1974 with the full battery of testing materials used in the laboratory for reading epilepsy. When these had been completed, he read books in which he was interested, particularly Indian lore, and throughout ten hours of observation there was no evidence either clinically or by EEG of seizures or seizure discharges. He was checked for the possibility of other types of reflex epilepsy, particularly in the visual sphere. The usual tests for photosensitivity, eye closure, and pattern-induced epilepsy were normal.

It was concluded that he had had reading epilepsy and that he had either had a spontaneous remission or he had found a technique for treating himself, that is, by completely avoiding reading for ten years.

CASE 2. This patient was a twenty-four-year-old auto assembly plant worker who had a single generalized major motor seizure in August of 1967 at age eighteen. The seizure occurred while reading. He noted jaw twitching during reading, and as he continued to read, the twitching increased in frequency. He then lost consciousness. During the seizure the patient fell, bit his tongue, and was unconscious for some three minutes after the seizure; upon awakening, he was confused.

In retrospect he had noted the association of jaw jerking with reading, which began several years prior to the occurrence of the major motor seizure. The jaw twitching would usually occur within five minutes after beginning to read, and if he stopped reading, the twitching disappeared. He noted that these episodes were more likely to occur with fatigue and lack of sleep and in the late afternoon. He did have them in the morning if he had had only a few hours of sleep.

Physical and neurological examinations were normal.

This patient was studied at the University of Wisconsin in 1968 and was definitely shown to have reading epilepsy. At that time he was not interested in pursuing any behavioral therapy, but returned to the Neurology Clinic six years later in February, 1974 for continued evaluation.

He was then studied in the Research Laboratory. His EEGs were normal in the routine and resting state, with hyperventilation, and during photic stimulation.

For five hours in the laboratory, he read the various types of material used in the complete battery for reading epilepsy. No dysrhythmia and no seizures occurred.

The patient then volunteered that he had done practically no reading other than the newspaper headlines for very short periods of time during the six years since the diagnosis of reading epilepsy had been made.

These two cases strongly suggest that the method of avoidance of stimulus can be employed in the treatment of reading epilepsy. However, for most of the patients described in Chapter 5, the price of this method of treatment would be too great since these seizures usually begin in adolescence. Avoidance of reading therefore would seriously interfere with education.

There are rare instances in reading epilepsy where the *partial avoidance of the stimulus* can be employed without interfering with life patterns. Case 9 (Chapter 5) had no seizures when reading quietly and could read for approximately five minutes aloud before experiencing a seizure. After his first study in the laboratory, when he understood these facts, he read quietly in unlimited amounts and limited his reading aloud to considerably less than five minutes. By following these principles, he was able to read aloud a short story to his children at bedtime and to participate in the services of his religion without evoking seizures. After three months of this training, his reading time before a seizure occurred had increased to ten minutes.

Thus a resourceful patient can employ the results of the careful laboratory studies and use them to further his seizure control and his life pursuits.

The *alteration of stimulus* is not usually feasible as a method for the treatment of reading epilepsy. The author and his colleagues have studied the effects of reading with various light intensities and the effect of changes in focus. This was accomplished by projecting the reading material upon a screen and out of focus, and gradually approaching clarity (or, in dim light, with gradual increases of illumination). When the material was readable, however, seizures occurred. Moreover, it was also noted that in all of the study patients, monocular reading evoked seizures just as readily as binocular.

An attempt at *stimulus alteration* was made in Case 1.[24] Since he had seizures only when reading aloud and not when reading quietly, the technique in this case consisted in having him read quietly for prolonged periods of time and then begin reading aloud. The period of time before seizure evocation could be extended somewhat by this technique. However, it was quite a cumbersome method.

The method of threshold alteration is characterized by repeated presentations in the postictal refractory state. This is impossible in reading epilepsy. The partial seizures are not followed by a postictal confusion or EEG slowing, therefore there is no refractory period. If the patient evoked a major motor seizure, the postictal confusion would prevent his reading, thus continuous presentations would not be possible during and immediately after the generalized major seizure.

Vigilance inhibition is the best method of behavioral treatment at the present time.[24, 25] It was noted in Chapter 5 that the patients with seizures reading digits did not have seizures when doing mathematical computations. Also, seizures did not occur when singing. This suggested that vigilance or concentration might abort the occurrence of seizures while reading.

A simple technique for employing the vigilance method consists of having the patient signal the occurrence of a particular letter. The signaling usually employed in the laboratory is having the patient press the thumb and forefinger of one hand together. The letter chosen is either a vowel or the consonants "s" and "t," since these commonly occur in the text. When this is done, most of the patients can read without the occurrence of seizures. One of the study patients (Case 2) read some five hundred pages of college text the weekend after his first five days of undergoing treatment in the laboratory. He found, however, that he had to change the signalled letter at approximately every fifty pages in order to maintain the effectiveness of the vigilance method.

The method of *avoidance conditioning* of course can play no role here, since the goal of therapy is to make it possible for the patient to read.

Decision-making Epilepsy

As yet the study has revealed no clues for a behavioral method of handling this type of epilepsy. It is obvious that the various methods mentioned, with the possible exception of vigilance, are not applicable. It is not possible to avoid decision making of the type which evokes the seizures; the nature of the stimulus precludes stimulus alteration, and the threshold alteration method cannot be employed.

Vigilance inhibition was attempted in Case 1 but was unsuccessful. Signalling the subjective occurrence of the seizures while playing chess did not prevent their occurrence. In a further attempt to explore the possible efficacy of vigilance, the patient was asked while playing chess to identify short portions of musical numbers played over the speaker system. He was also asked to whistle a particular tune over and over, during which the author listened, correcting him for errors. In all of these situations, the seizures evoked by playing chess still occurred. At the present time, no behavioral methods of therapy have been developed for this form of reflex epilepsy. This type of epilepsy might be considered as relevant to Pavlov's production of experimental neurosis in the dog by a difficult discrimination.

Somatosensory-Evoked Epilepsy

The *avoidance of the evoking stimulus* is impossible in either the simple or the complex form of somatosensory-evoked epilepsy. The inadvertent tap by bumping into an object, the affectionate gesture of a child or sibling, or the jolt in the course of play readily evokes seizures in the simple type of somatosensory-evoked epilepsy.

In the complex type, the rubbing stimulus also cannot always be avoided. Case 3 in Chapter 7, when picking up and rolling up some architectural designs upon conclusion of a business meeting, had them unfurl and rub against the palmar surface of his left wrist, and a seizure occurred. In Case 4, ablutions involving face washing, hair combing, and toothbrushing evoked seizures. Obviously, none of these grooming and health care activities can be avoided.

The *stimulus alteration* method is effective in the treatment of the simple type of somatosensory-evoked epilepsy. The unilateral presentation method of alteration cannot be used because of the unilaterality of the reflexogenous zones. The alteration of the stimulus, however, can be achieved in the intensity or location of the stimulus. The tap can be applied so lightly as not to evoke the dysrhythmia and then gradually be increased in intensity far beyond that necessary to evoke a seizure.

These patients also have a specific, well-defined area of the body which is reflexogenous. In Case 1, this involved the left shoulder and in Case 2, the right thigh and epigastrium. The stimulus can be administered outside the reflexogenous zone and gradually administered closer and closer until it enters the zone.

When the stimulus is administered repeatedly in either of these altered forms and without evoking a dysrhythmia, there is a refractory period, or a period of time during which the reflex seizures cannot be elicited by appropriate stimuli. This at first is a matter of a minute or less, but with repeated presentations of the altered stimulus, the duration can be extended. Case 1 was studied many years ago (long before the author became involved in behavioral concepts). Reviewing in 1974 the films made of the patient in 1948 shows both of these effects, stimulus alteration in intensity and in location. This is an example, at that time (1948), of looking and not seeing!

The conditioned response is specific for the type of stimulus. In Case 2, since the seizures could be evoked by electric shocks to the skin as well as by tapping, the laboratory physicians felt that it would be simpler to use skin shocks for the conditioning. These could be controlled at a distance, without the patient having any ability to determine the time of their possible administration and, moreover, were more easily controlled for strength of stimulus than were manually administered taps. However, when the patient had been treated with skin shocks of gradually increasing intensity and no longer had seizures evoked by the shocks, a brisk tap to the reflexogenous zone immediately evoked a seizure. Therefore, no generalization to tactile stimuli occurred from the electric skin shocks.

In the simple type, *alteration of threshold* obtained by the utilization of a postictal refractory phase is not possible. The seizures are of the short, brief, absence variety and are not followed by a postictal phase.

In the complex type, however, the threshold alteration can be employed. In Case 4, Chapter 7, it was impossible to induce a seizure in the laboratory after the EEG electrode placement had served as an evoking stimulus. In Case 3, Chapter 7, the patient had himself learned to employ the refractory period. Each morning, before leaving the house, he would induce a psychomotor type of seizure by stimulating his left palm. The refractory period which this induced lasted for the rest of the day. This then is an unusual example of the use of the postictal refractory phase as a form of self-induced epilepsy, but with a definite purpose, namely the therapeutic prevention, for the duration of the day, of seizures inadvertently evoked by tactile stimuli.

Vigilance inhibition would be impossible to employ in the simple type of somatosensory-evoked epilepsy, and, in the study cases, had no effect in the complex type.

Avoidance conditioning obviously plays no role.

Reflex Epilepsy Related to Eating

Avoidance of the evoking stimulus is impossible because the patients cannot avoid eating. Case 2 did attempt this to some extent by severe fasting which represented a partial avoidance of the evoking stimulus. However, this failed to have any effect upon the course of her illness. It is not possible to continue complete avoidance of the stimulus for the periods of time noted for musicogenic and reading epilepsy (a matter of years).

Stimulus alteration also was not possible. The precise stimulus was never sharply defined despite all laboratory efforts. Stimulus alteration could not be applied to changes in food temperature, texture, or taste. However, in attempts at stimulus alteration, the duration of stimulation was changed. It seemed in the early part of the studies that the patient's seizures occurred after eating for at least three minutes. It therefore seemed logical to attempt to treat her by having her eat for one to two minute intervals, then stop for five minutes, and then again resume eating. During this period of tentative treatment she had a seizure at the very beginning of one of her meals, and on close questioning, it was found this had happened before.

The method of *threshold alteration* also could not be employed. The patient undoubtedly had a postictal refractory period but could not continue the stimulus (eating) because of the paralysis of face, tongue, pharynx, and larynx. Once she had recovered, she could continue to eat and did not have a second seizure during the meal. For this reason, she was instructed to chew gum continuously, with an ample quid between meals, in the hope of continuing whatever refractory period she may have acquired from her seizure at breakfast. This, however, was not successful, for she had a seizure at the next meal.

The *vigilance inhibition* method was found to be the most successful. The patient was given a counting device such as is used in hematology laboratories for cell counts. She was instructed to press the plunger at the initiation of each swallow so that during the meal each swallow was accounted for. She was observed closely for errors. If she failed to keep an accurate count, the AV tape was replayed to demonstrate to her the occurrence of the errors.

Seizures Evoked by Movement

In the patient with seizures induced by movement, no detailed behavioral therapeutic studies were made. Since she was in school, it was necessary to complete the observations as quickly as possible. Also, adequate doses of anticonvulsant medication, as noted in Chapter 14, controlled her seizures.

If this remission with medication had not occurred, it was planned to restudy her during the summer vacation. Since the seizures could be so readily evoked by suggestion, it was felt that behavioral therapy based on suggestion might have a beneficial effect.

Table XVI presents a summary of the applications of the various behavioral methods to the specific forms of reflex epilepsy. It should be noted that avoidance of the stimulus, either voluntarily or as a result of avoidance conditioning, is of very limited use. Avoidance of the stimulus is only efficacious in reading epilepsy and in musicogenic epilepsy, and then under unusual circumstances. The very nature of the evoking stimulus in reflex

TABLE XVI

Methods of behavioral therapy	Visually induced				Auditory-evoked					Somatosensory			
	Photic	Pattern	Eye closure	Color/object	Simple	Complex	Musico-genic	Reading	Decision	Simple	Complex	Eating	Movement
Avoidance of stimulus													
Complete	I	I	I	?	I	I	(+)	+	I	I	I	I	I
Partial	I	I	I	?	I	I	(+)	+	I	I	I	I	I
Stimulus alteration													
Unilateral presentation	+	+	+	0	+	0	0	0	0	0	0	I	I
Altered intensity	+	+	+	0	+	0	0	0	0	+	0	I	?
Without startle	-	-	-	-	+	0	0	0	0	+	0	I	?
Other	?	+	?	0	0	0	+	+	0	+	0	0	?
Threshold alteration	0	0	0	+	0	+	+	I	I	0	+	I	0
Vigilance inhibition	I	I	I	I	I	I	I	+	0	0	I	+	?
Avoidance conditioning	?	?	I	+	I	I	I	0	I	I	I	I	I

I – Impossible to use
+ – Effective
0 – Ineffective
? – Insufficient evidence
( ) – From cases in literature

Case numbers refer to Table II in Chap. 2.

epilepsy usually precludes the use of stimulus avoidance. The avoidance conditioning has a very limited usefulness but could be employed in patients with self-induction of seizures, when such self-induction is not for the purpose of preventing subsequent seizures.

The method of stimulus alteration is primarily useful in the simple types of reflex epilepsy. The item "other" under the category of stimulus alteration in Table XVI refers in pattern epilepsy to alterations of focus, in musicogenic epilepsy to the admixture of nonevoking and evoking renditions of the musical numbers, and in the simple form of somatosensory-evoked epilepsy to the presentation of stimuli outside the reflexogenous zones and moving into it.

A question mark under "other" kinds of stimulus alteration in the column on photosensitivity indicates that there may be ways of modifying the stimulus other than those which the study has tried. The other question marks indicate insufficient evidence from the studies in two rare cases, viz. the color/object-induced epilepsy and the patient with movement-induced epilepsy.

This chapter has discussed the various kinds of behavioral therapy and their application to the particular forms and types of reflex epilepsy. In general it would seem that the repeated presentation of the altered evoking stimulus is the most effective method for the behavioral therapy in the simple types of reflex epilepsy. The use of the postictal refractory phase contains the most effective method for the behavioral treatment of complex forms when the patient does not control the stimulus presentation. It should be noted that these two methods dealing with the intensity of the evoking stimulus and the level of seizure threshold have basic similarities, as they deal with reciprocal relationships.

The term "behavioral" is used to include the entire gamut of these therapeutic approaches. The methods vary from simple, voluntary, behavioral expression on the part of the patient, to operant conditioning. The conscious avoidance of the evoking stimulus, when feasible, is a simple behavioral approach on the part of the patient. By contrast, the administration of skin shock stimuli when the patient seeks out the evoking stimulus, with the resultant avoidance of the evoking stimulus, is operant conditioning.

Between these two extremes of behavioral methods are the other methods which have been described. The author and his colleagues have come to consider these, namely stimulus alterations and threshold alterations, as conditioning processes. The controlled systematic and repeated presentations of the stimulus results in the establishment of a learning process, albeit unconsciously, within the central nervous system. This learning process yields predictable results.

The data were reviewed early in the course of these studies by Doctor W. Horsley Gantt, and he concluded that this is indeed a conditioning process, albeit different from other known methods of conditioning.

REFERENCES

1. Servit, Z.: *Reflex Mechanisms in the Genesis of Epilepsy*. Amsterdam, London, New York, Elsevier, 1963.
2. Forster, F. M. and Bennett, D. R.: Reading epilepsy. *Electroencephalogr Clin Neurophysiol, 33*:240, 1972.
3. Shaw, D. and Hill, D.: A case of musicogenic epilepsy. *J Neurol Neurosurg Psychiat, 10*:107, 1947.
4. Forster, F. M.: Conditional reflexes and sensory-evoked epilepsy: The nature of the therapeutic process. *Cond Reflex, 4*:103, 1969.
5. Jung, R.: Blocking of petit mal attacks by sensory arousal and inhibition of attacks by an active change in attention during the epileptic aura. *Epilepsia, 3*:435, 1962.
6. Cleeland, C. S. and Booker, H. E.: Petit mal evoked by arousal during sensory restriction. *Arch Neurol, 17*:324, 1967.
7. Tassinari, C. A.: Suppresion of focal spikes by somato-sensory stimuli. *Electroencephalogr Clin Neurophysiol, 25*:574, 1969.
8. Prince, D. A.: Modification of focal cortical epileptogenic discharges by afferent impulses. *Epilepsia, 7*:181, 1966.
9. Chocholova, L.: Epileptic attacks and adaptation. *Epilepsia, 3*:350- 1962.
10. Efron, R.: Conditioning inhibition of uncinate fits. *Brain, 80*:251, 1957.
11. Sterman, M. B. and Friar, L.: Suppression of seizures in an epileptic following sensorimotor feedback EEG training. *Electroencephalogr Clin Neurophysiol, 33*:89, 1972.
12. Sterman, M. D., MacDonald, L. R., and Stone, R. K.: Biofeedback

training of sensorimotor cortex EEG in man and its effects upon epilepsy. *Electroencephaogr Clin Neurophysiol,* 25:574, 1968.

13. Wyler, A. R., Fetz, E. E., and Ward, A. A.: Effects of operant conditioning epileptic unit activity on seizure frequencies and electrophysiologic of neocortical experimenteal foci. *Exp Neurol,* 44:113, 1974.

15. Forster, F. M., Ptacek, L. J., and Peterson, W. G.: Auditory clicks in extinction of stroboscope-induced seizures. *Epilepsia,* 6:217, 1965.

16. Forster, F. M. and Booker, H. E.: Conditioning therapy in photosensitive seizures. *Trans Am Neurol Assoc,* 93:99, 1968.

17. Forster, F. M.: Conditioning of cerebral dysrhythmia induced by pattern presentation and eye closure. *Cond Reflex,* 2:236, 1967.

18. Booker, H. E., Forster, F. M., and Klove, H.: Extinction factors in startle (acousticomotor) seizures. *Neurology,* 15:1095, 1965.

19. Forster, F. M., Cleeland, G., Hansotia, P., and Ludwig, A.: A case of voice induced epilepsy treated by conditioning. *Neurology,* 19:325, 1969.

20. Titeca, J.: L'epilepsie musicogenique. Rev. general à propros un cas pse personnel. *Acta Neurol Belg,* 65:598, 1965.

21. Forster, F. M., Klove, H., Peterson, W. G., and Bengzon, A. R. A.: Modification of musicogenic epilepsy by extinction technique. *Trans Am Neurol Assoc,* 90:179, 1965.

22. Szabor, A. and Frater, R.: Contributions to the study of musicogenic epilepsy. *Ther Hung,* 4:8, 1955.

23. Forster, F. M., Booker, H. E., and Gascon, G.: Conditioning in musicogenic epilepsy. *Trans Am Neurol Assoc,* 92:236, 1967.

24. Forster, F. M., Paulsen, W. A., and Baughman, F. A.: Clinical therapeutic conditioning in reading epilepsy. *Neurology,* 19:717, 1969.

CHAPTER 13

BEHAVIORAL THERAPY OF REFLEX EPILEPSY: MAINTENANCE OR REINFORCEMENT OF THERAPY

T HE RESEARCH LABORATORY's earliest clinical studies in reflex epilepsy were carried out on patients with photosensitivity. In the first patient, a reinforcement technique (as described below) was inadvertently employed. Not until the second patient was studied and followed did those involved with the study realize the necessity of developing methods for reinforcement or main-tenance of the conditioned effect when the patients were treated with the stimulus alteration techniques. With this experience in the patients with photosensitivity, it could then be assumed that reinforcement would also be necessary in other forms of reflex epilepsy. Therefore methods were developed which were especially applicable for the patients treated for other forms of reflex epilepsy such as musicogenic and voice-induced. Sub-sequent observations in Chapter 15 show that this premise was correct. In this chapter, the various methods employed for reinforcement are described.

VISUALLY INDUCED EPILEPSY

The first patient (Case 1, Chapter 2), a University student, was adjusting her television for "flop-over" when she stated "I feel funny" and had a convulsion. When studied in the labora-tory, she was found on photic stimulation to be photosensitive between fifteen and thirty-five cycles per second. This stimula-tion evoked an atypical wave and spike dysrhythmia associated with a myoclonic jerk. She then volunteered that she had had this type of seizure—a myoclonic jerk—whenever she passed a picket fence in the sunlight or in similar circumstances. Because of her class schedule, the amount of time she could spend in the laboratory was limited. Accordingly, each Saturday morning was set aside for an attempt at treatment. It had been noted in the laboratory that monocular presentations evoked no dysrhyhmia. Therefore, she was given repeated monocular presentations, first to one eye, then to the other. Because of the limited laboratory time, she was instructed after the first session, at home each night, to patch one eye with a velvet patch and kneel in front of the TV set exactly as she had been doing when she suffered her first major seizure. Her husband (an engineer) produced a flop-over effect at approximately the same frequencies. This was done for ten to fifteen minute intervals each night to each eye. Thus, quite accidentally, the principle of maintenance or reinforcement of the conditioning was introduced.

The second patient (Case 2, Chapter 2) had four to forty minor seizures per day and occasional major motor seiures. Some of her seizures were self-induced and evoked by hand waving while looking at a bright light. This was often done to avoid unpleasant chores in the home.

Monocular presentations were tried as the method of treatment, but the patient became fatigued and allowed her hand holding the velvet patch to slip. This led to inadvertent light leaks into the eye with vision presumably occluded. Thus she developed monocular sensitivity. Cases 2 and 3, Chapter 2, were being studied concurrently. Case 3, with only one eye, was of course monocularly sensitive. Interest in this patient led to the development of the differential light intensity treatment. Because of the difficulty of maintaining monocular presentations, the differential light intensity technique was also employed in Case 2. Her sensitivity to intermittent light could be markedly decreased or abolished in laboratory sessions of one to two hours. However, this was short lived, and the seizures recurred at home.

The first attempts at reinforcement consisted in weekly sessions of two and one-half to three hours each. It was possible to reduce or abolish her photosensitivity each Sunday, but during the week the seizures recurred. After several months it was obvious that no real control of seizures was being accomplished by the weekly reinforcement sessions. Daily sessions in the laboratory were not feasible so it was decided to test another possibility, that is, whether or not a second-signal system would prevent the occurrence of seizures after the conditioning process.

In the laboratory, earphones were put in place on the patient. The earphones were activated by a photoelectric cell. When the flashes of light at the appropriate intensity were presented and coupled with clicks, seizures and dysrhythmia occurred. Therefore, the audible clicks triggered by the photoelectric cells in themselves would not inhibit the occurrence of the seizures.[1]

The patient was then given a course of therapy using the differential light intensity technique. Each flash of light was accompanied by a simultaneous click. After three sessions in the laboratory, the light intensity could be brought to the point which previously evoked seizures, but without the occurrence of a dysrhythmia or seizure (Fig. 65). If, however, the photoelectric cell was covered and she was again administered the same visual stimulation, but now without the accompanying auditory click, the dysrhythmia and seizure occurred (Figs. 66, 67). Uncovering the cell immediately afterwards, and administering the same light stimulation coupled with a simultaneous click, prevented the occurrence of the dysrhythmia and seizure. This study showed that adding a second-signal system in the auditory sphere to the differential light intensity treatment method could prevent the occurrence of seizures.

The earphone-photoelectric cell combination was too cumbersome and impractical for daily use. Therefore, a special pair of eyeglasses was devised. These glasses have a photoelectric cell over the bridge of the nose which by special circuitry activates a hearing aid device over the mastoid on one side. Each time there is a flash of light, a click timed exactly with the light flash is audible to the patient.

Patients were treated by the differential light intensity technique wearing these glasses throughout the process. During the course of the treatment, the patients received over a million audible clicks associated with visual stimuli which, because of the altered stimulus technique, had failed to evoke dysrhythmias. For example, the patients who were stimulated at twenty cycles

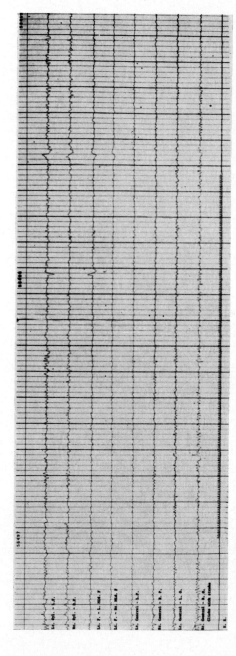

Figure 65. Effect of second-signal system in preventing photic-induced dysrhythmia. (Case 2, Chapter 2.) Photoelectric cell activating earphones. After conditioning, photic driving but no evoked dysrhythmia. Reprinted from *Epilepsia*, 6:217, 1965.

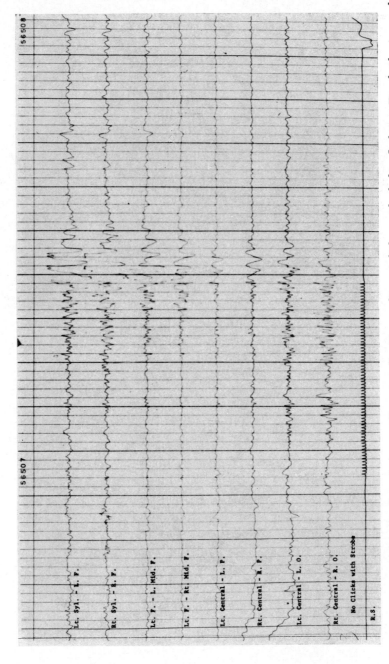

Figure 66. Same patient. Photoelectric cell covered. No auditory clicks with light flashes. Dysrhythmia evoked. Reprinted from *Epilepsia*, 6:217, 1965.

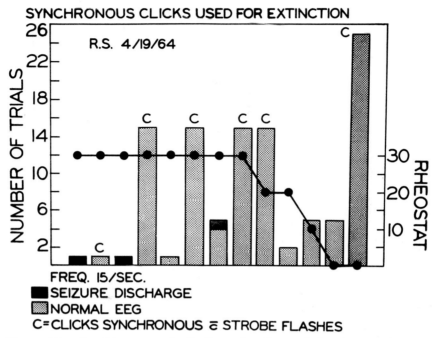

SYNCHRONOUS CLICKS USED FOR EXTINCTION

FREQ. 15/SEC.
- ■ SEIZURE DISCHARGE
- ▧ NORMAL EEG
- C= CLICKS SYNCHRONOUS c̄ STROBE FLASHES

Figure 67. Graphic portrayal of effect of auditory clicks after conditioning procedure. No dysrhythmia evoked by flashing light when coupled with auditory clicks after conditioning has taken place. Reprinted from *Epilepsia*, 6:217, 1965.

per second, received 1,200 stimulations per minute or 72,000 per hour. Since the patients spent approximately five hours per day and had ten days of treatment in the two week interval, this is equivalent to 1.8 million pairs of innocuous visual stimuli and auditory clicks.

The special glasses served two purposes. The first and most important was that they gave the patients, in their day-to-day environment, protection by the second-signal system. The glasses also served as a means of day-to-day reinforcement of the conditioning process. The patients, throughout their normal routine (riding in a car, walking along the street), were exposed to frequent changes in light stimulation, and each was accompanied by a protective audible click.

Figure 68 shows the specially designed eyeglasses used in this form of maintenance or reinforcement of therapy. The

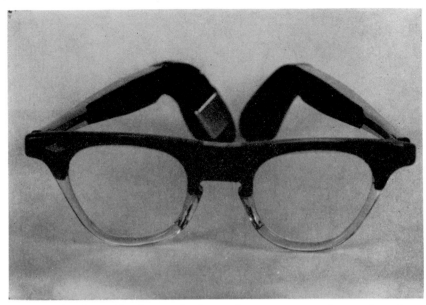

Figure 68. Specially designed glasses for patients conditions for photo-sensitivity. Over the bridge of the nose is a photoelectric cell, connected to the hearing aid device over the mastoid process. Each flash of light is accompanied by an audible click. (Glasses compliments of Otarion Hearing Aid.) Reprinted from *Epilepsia, 6*:217, 1965.

process of converting variations in light intensity into audible sounds is more complicated than simply connecting a photocell to an earphone. The problems involved along with their solutions are discussed below in reference to the circuit shown in Figure 69.[1]

The device is capable of proper operation under any normal ambient lighting condition, from a dimly lighted room to bright sunny day outdoors. This is accomplished, for the moment neglecting the filter made up of R_2, R_3, R_4, C_1, C_2, and C_3, by using a cadmium sulfate photocell (photoconductive) Ph_1 and a resistor R_1 in a voltage divider and a capactitor C_4. As the light intensity increases on the photocell, the voltage across R_1 decreases. C_4 will allow only the rapid changes in voltage caused by rapid changes in light intensity on the photocell to pass on to the next stage and block the slower changing or DC voltages caused by ambient light.

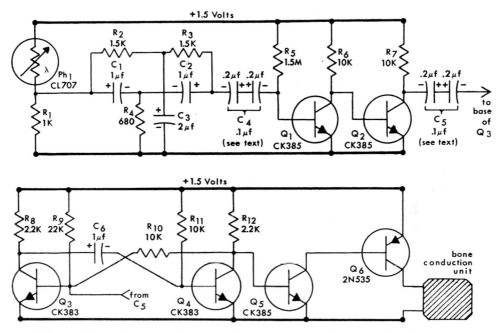

Figure 69. Schema or diagram for circuitry in the specially designed glasses in Figure 68. Reprinted from *Epilepsia,* 6:217, 1965.

The photocell used, unfortunately, will respond to the peaks of light present in fluorescent lighting. Even though these peaks cannot be seen, they can cause an interference that would disrupt the operation of the entire device. This interference is eliminated by use of the filter mentioned above, a double T filter whose values were calculated to eliminate the 120 cycle interference caused by the peaks present in 60 cycle fluorescent light. If interference caused by such lighting operated on other power line frequencies is to be eliminated, different component values must be used in the filter.

The frequency of the light variations which are of interest are below the audible range when converted to acoustical power. They can be made audible, however, in the form of "clicks," by electronically converting each cycle into a uniform square pulse of voltage with a fast rise time and a duration of approximately 10 msec. These pulses are generated by the single-shot multivibrators Q_3 and Q_4. C_6 and R_{11} determine the pulse duration.

It is triggered by the voltage changes developed across R_1 which have been filtered, differentiated (C_4 and input of Q_3), and amplified, and limited in height by Q_1 and Q_2. The pulses from the multivibrator are then amplified by Q_5 and Q_6 to give them sufficient power to drive the bone conduction unit.

The components used are all subminiature hearing aid types. The resistors are all Ohmite® "Little Devil" 0.1 watt, 10 per cent carbon. The capacitors are Ohmite series TW tantalum wire capacitors. This type of capacitor is polarized, and therefore a reverse voltage should not be allowed across it. In the case of C_4 and C_5, the voltage across them will reverse in normal operation. By connecting them back to back, as shown, they will act as nonpolarized capacitors because one will prevent a reverse voltage from being applied across the other. The photocell is manufactured by the Clairex Corporation, transistors Q_1 through Q_5 are Raytheon, and Q_6 is Philco. The bone conduction unit is built into the eyeglass frame which is manufactured by Otarion. A silver oxide cell is used as the power source in preference to a mercury cell, because its voltage is higher initially (1.5 V compared to 1.4 V for mercury) and is more constant over its operating life.

Patients with less severe photosensitivity were treated in the laboratory with repeated monocular presentations. For maintenance or reinforcement of the conditioning, these patients were given portable stroboscopes to take home and were instructed to treat themselves two or three times a day. The stimulations in these periods were all administered monocularly, and the patients were carefully advised to place the patch over one eye before turning on the stroboscope. They were also cautioned to turn off the stimulus before either moving the patch from one eye to the other or removing the patch at the conclusion of the session. The stimulations were carried out for ten to fifteen minutes to each eye in the morning and evening and, if feasible, depending upon the patients' school schedules, also at noon. In Case 1, the use of television adjusted for flop-over served the same function for monocular presentations.

These two forms of reinforcement or maintenance therapy are quite different. The patients treated with monocular stimulations, who are maintaining the conditioned effect by daily repeated monocular stimulations represent a very simple and direct kind of reinforcement.

However, the patients wearing the specially designed eyeglasses are employing a different phenomenon. This is a true second-signal conditioning system. The auditory clicks are not able to prevent the seizures before conditioning therapy, but after the multiple presentations of light flashes without the evocation of seizures, auditory clicks have acquired a protective and reinforcing function.

The patients with pattern epilepsy who have been conditioned, and in whom success in maintaining the conditioning has been achieved, have also been photosensitive. In all cases except Case 27, conditioning was paired; that is, the patterns were presented on the screen at the same time as the stroboscopic stimulations and using the differential light intensity method. This treatment is equally effective for pattern epilepsy and photosensitivity. Case 27 (Chapter 2) was treated separately. These patients in their day-to-day environment are, of course, wearing the special glasses. Sample patterns, both the ones which precipitated seizures and/or dysrhythmia and some of the patterns which did not, were given to the patients to take home. Two or three times a day, they were instructed to stare at the patterns while finger waving in front of the glasses so as to couple the clicks due to intermittent light with the viewing of the patterns.

AUDITORY-EVOKED EPILEPSY

For the simple type of auditory evoked epilepsy, a reinforcement method was recently developed in the Research Laboratory. Unfortunately, many of the patients with startle epilepsy are quite retarded, and their lack of cooperation hinders the process. At first, special audio tapes were made which recorded all the evoking sounds presented during the laboratory conditioning sessions. To these tapes were also added sounds which had been known to evoke seizures in the patient's home and which had also been used in the laboratory. The tapes were played by the family to the patient several times a day in an attempt

to maintain the conditioning process. This did not prove successful, probably because here the simple type of reflex epilepsy,
treated by stimulus alteration in contrast to the threshold
alteration method, was involved.

In the laboratory a technique was recently developed for
administering a second-signal system for the reinforcement of
the therapy for the simple type of auditory-evoked epilepsy.[2]
This consists of a small pack which can be carried on the person
(Fig. 70), for example in a shirt pocket. Environmental sounds
are detected by a microphone, then amplified and rectified by
an absolute value amplifier, producing a DC voltage change
proportional to the ambient sound level. An automatic gain
control on the amplifier helps to maintain a stable output voltage.

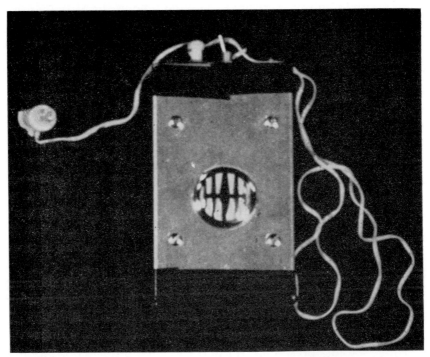

Figure 70. Second-signal system device for acousticomotor epilepsy.
Microphone on face of pack picks up ambient noises. Hearing aid is
placed in ear of patient. Each alteration of ambient noise level is signalled to patient by a "beep" transmitted through the hearing aid.

Changes in this voltage, reflecting sudden or abrupt noises, are detected by a circuit which triggers a tone if the rate of change in the voltage is greater than a present value (internally adjustable). When the circuit is triggered, a brief tone is generated and fed to the patient's earphone. Both the volume and duration of the tone may be adjusted by the patient. The pack is so designed that it picks up increments in ambient noises; a constant steady noise is only perceived at its onset. Any additional noise above this ambient level is also picked up by the sensordevice. The device sends a signal, in the form of a "beep," within the type of hearing aid.

In the treatment of the photosensitive patients, the second-signal system device involves a different sensory system. The first signal is visual (a flashing light), and the second signal is auditory. There was some concern that it might not be possible in startle epilepsy to use the same system, that is, an auditory signal for both the first and second signal. However, it has proven feasible. This method is relatively new and has not yet been applied to the forms of auditory-evoked epilepsy other than the startle or acousticomotor types. In order to be certain that there is adequate startle stimulation each day to maintain the conditioning, the patients are also supplied with an audio tape of the evoked sounds from the laboratory, and these are played to the patient at home twice a day (of course, while the patient is wearing the device).

A different technique was employed in the complex types of auditory-evoked epilepsy, for example that induced by specific voices and in musicogenic epilepsy. In the course of behavioral therapy, when a specific voice or music stimulus had evoked a seizure and the altered threshold had been used for therapy, this evoking sound was placed on an audio tape. The patient subsequently took this tape (designated as his master tape) to his/her hospital room and listened to the tape repeatedly during the day. As the process of treatment continued, each additional voice or musical number which had evoked a seizure or dys-rhythmia was added to the tape after the repeated presentation.

In both voice-induced and in musicogenic epilepsy, since the seizures were evoked in the sleeping state, it was also possible to use the sleep state for maintenance of conditioning. This was especially important in two of the patients with musicogenic epilepsy whose tapes required about an hour and a half of listening, twice a day. By using an alarm clock-radio device, it was possible to have their tapes turned off after they had gone to sleep or turned on in the morning before they awakened so that a large part of this three-hour time could transpire without interfering with their daily routine.

READING EPILEPSY

While the conditioning therapy in reading epilepsy leaves much to be desired, there is no doubt that the vigilance technique does play a role in controlling the occurrence of the seizures. Usually there is no need for reinforcement. If, however, reinforcement is necessary, there is a very simple way to accomplish this. As noted, all but one of the eleven study patients with reading epilepsy had no difficulties reading memorized material. If the signalling of the vowel or consonant loses its efficacy, it is possible to reconstitute this by reading safe material, i.e. material memorized by the patient, as the twenty-third Psalm, the Lord's Prayer, or the Gettysburg Address, while signalling the occurrence of certain letters. It has been noted in the laboratory that this again makes the vigilance technique effective.

SOMATOSENSORY EPILEPSY

Maintenance conditioning was attempted in only one of the four patients with somatosensory evoked epilepsy. This was in Case 2, Chapter 7, the young lady with seizures evoked by a brisk tap to the right thigh or lower abdomen. A special switching device was designed for her to wear over her thigh. Upon contact with the device (two filamentous plates encased in plastic), the plates came in contact with each other, closed a circuit and delivered a click in a hearing aid device over the right mastoid. She was instructed daily to tap briskly and repeatedly upon this switching device so as to have a series of safe stimulations with' audible clicks. It should be noted that she was not able to elicit a seizure by self-stimulation unless it was accidental and inadvertent. Thus the conscious stimulation of the reflexogenous zone would not evoke seizures. This, therefore, provided a method for giving simple, safe stimulations to reinforce the prior conditioning effect.

In the cooperative patient with seizures associated with eating, no reinforcement was necessary since the vigilance method with each meal sufficed.

In summary, in epilepsy associated with eating and usually in reading epilepsy, reinforcement is not necessary. In these instances, the patients are in control of the stimulus presentation and can couple this with vigilance techniques.

In the other forms of reflex epilepsy described, the treatment, while successful in the laboratory phase, requires repeated reinforcement. This can be accomplished in some cases by a daily repeating of the laboratory experience. This is seen in the patients with monocular, stroboscopic presentations as well as in the patients listening daily to the music or voices which evoked their seizures. A second-signal system, however, is necessary for many patients. This has been successfully devised for the photosensitive patients and for certain of the simple auditory-induced epilepsies.

REFERENCES

1. Forster, F. M., Ptacek, L. J., and Peterson, W. G.: Auditory clicks in extinction of stroboscope-induced seizures. *Epilepsia,* 6:217, 1965.
2. Forster, F. M. and Harley, J. P.: Use of a second signal system in the conditioning therapy of acoustico-motor epilepsy. *Neurology,* 25: 361, 1975.

CHAPTER 14

BEHAVIORAL THERAPY OF REFLEX EPILEPSY: SELECTION OF CASES AND ROLE OF MEDICATION

As will be shown in the next chapter, behavioral therapy can be successfully employed in the treatment of reflex epilepsy. However, as is obvious from the preceding two chapters, the process can be long and demanding in time for both the investigator and the patient, or his family, and requires diligent attention after the laboratory process when the patient has returned home. Therefore, case selection is important. The following are the most important criteria in case selection for behavioral therapy.

DEFINITE EVIDENCE THAT SEIZURES ARE REFLEX IN NATURE

The seizures must be reflex in nature if these methods of behavioral therapy are to be successful. The criteria for the diagnosis of reflex epilepsy have been reviewed in the earlier chapters in this book. In essence, reflex epilepsy consists of the predictable evocation of specific seizures upon the presentation of specific stimuli.

Some patients with reflex epilepsy, however, have a mixture of stimulus-induced and spontaneous seizures. This may complicate the treatment process, especially in photosensitive patients when computer automation is being considered for therapy. It is not possible for the computer to differentiate between spontaneous and sensory evoked dysrhythmias; thus the computer can be repeatedly triggered by the spontaneous dysrhythmia. The preliminary recordings in the sensory-deprived state allow the laboratory to obtain a baseline for the amount of dysrhythmia which occurs independent of auditory or visual input. The presence of one or two bursts of dysrhythmia in the time period of the sensory-deprived state does not exclude the patient from the conditioning process. But any substantial amount of non-evoked dysrhythmia, with the possible resultant interruptions of the conditioning process, suggests that the patient is not a candidate for this form of therapy, particularly when computer automation is to be used.

As has been noted before, multiple types of sensory-evoked epilepsy may occur in the same patient. This does not necessarily rule out the possibility of behavioral treatment of the patient by the conditioning process. Patients with both photo-sensitivity and pattern epilepsy can be treated, and the two conditions can be handled simultaneously. If the need arises, the two conditions, namely photosensitivity and pattern epilepsy, can also be treated independently. For example, Case 27, Chapter 2, was photosensitive and was successfully treated in the laboratory. But despite reinforcement with the glasses, she continued to have some seizures. These seizures were found to be pattern-evoked. The pattern-evoked seizures were also treated by conditioning therapy. It should be noted that this patient also had some spontaneous discharges and seizures, but these did not interfere with the conditioning process for either the photic or pattern sensitivity forms.

FREQUENCY AND SEVERITY OF SEIZURES

In a given patient, the reflex epilepsy must be a severe enough problem to warrant institution of behavioral therapy. A patient with a rare seizure is not a subject for the prolonged treatment process, nor is the patient whose photosensitivity is limited to a dysrhythmia but without clinical seizures. The incidence and/or severity of seizures should be great enough to warrant undergoing therapy.

The history of the occurrence of generalized major motor seizures by light stimulation certainly warrants the use of behavioral therapy if other methods have failed. Such a history would include seizures when looking at the sea or a similar body of moving water, or on self-induction of seizures by hand waving. When daily minor seizures or the occurrence of repeated major motor seizures are present, there is an adequate indication of severity and frequency to warrant behavioral therapy. As in the consideration of any form of therapy the particular condition of the patient is also important. Various physical and psychological factors have to be taken into consideration. These include occupational hazards, the responsibility on the part of the patient for the well-being of others, as well as the social and psychological impact of the seizure disorder upon the patient.

SEIZURES AS PART OF A PROGRESSIVE DISEASE

The presence of a progressive disease associated with the seizures makes it difficult to obtain satisfactory results. In the study cases of progressive cerebellar myoclonus with photosensitivity, for example, transient improvement was obtained by the therapeutic pocess but the progressive course of the disease made any satisfactory long-term result impossible. The gains accomplished by the treatment were offset by the progressive degeneration of the patient.

INTELLIGENCE AND MOTIVATION

Intelligence is not an important factor in the first stage of therapy. It may, however, play a role in the process of reinforcement or maintenance of therapy especially after the patient has left the hospital. The patient with the greatest retardation in the study series (Case 3, Chapter 2), with trisomy-D anomaly and photosensitivity, could, by the differential light intensity technique, be rendered insensitive to flashing lights for a period of several hours. But it was not possible or feasible to employ the reinforcement method with any success.

Motivation to guarantee cooperation is not a serious problem in the first stage of therapy for photosensitive or acousticomotor epilepsy. The stimulus can be administered to the patient in the laboratory with little or no cooperation. Pattern epilepsy, however, presents a different situation. If the young child will not view the patterns during the treatment sessions, nothing can be accomplished.

However, on occasion, a patient with certain features of visually induced epilepsy, because of insufficient cooperation and motivation, cannot be carried through the altered stimulus phases of the clinical therapeutic conditioning. An example of this was a child who, as a special feature, was photosensitive only with her eyes open. She would not keep her eyes open during the computer automation steps. She would close them at the higher light level and would suddenly open them at times when the ambient room light decreased to low levels. This would immediately evoke a seizure because she had not had the benefit of the gradual decreases in light intenesity with her eyes open.

Cooperation and motivation are of greatest importance in the maintenance or reinforcement of the conditioning process. It is necessary for the patient, on a daily basis, to maintain the conditioned state over a sufficient period of time, usually several years. Failure to do so will invariably lead to a return of seizures. In the younger patients, the cooperation of the parents is necessary to maintain the reinforcement procedure. If the parents and/or the patient are incapable or unwilling to extend themselves, then the entire procedure is valueless.

ROLE OF ANTIEPILEPTIC MEDICATIONS

Obviously it is much simpler, and less time consuming, if the patient can be successfully treated with antiepileptic medications. This is also somewhat less dependent upon continued cooperation of the patient. The taking of medication is less demanding in time and effort than is the continuation of the reinforcement methods.

In some of the patients described herein, the antiepileptic medications succeeded in establishing complete seizure control: The patient with seizures evoked by movement of her right arm (Case 1, Chapter 9) was studied for possible behavioral therapy. It was assumed that adequate dosages of diphenylhydantoin and phenobarbital prescribed for her had failed to control her seizures. However, on admission, her serum blood levels for these medications were extremely low. When confronted with this she admitted that she had not been taking her medications. When these were administered in the hospital, the serum levels rose to therapeutic levels and the seizures disappeared. She had two Jacksonian seizures in the succeeding seven months.

The patient with seizures evoked by decision making (Case 1, Chapter 6) was given adequate doses of diphenylhydantoin and primidone, as determined by blood levels. He was then engaged in decision making for four hours without the occurrence of seizures or evoked dysrhythmias. This far surpassed the time period needed prior to medication for the evocation of seizures. Fortunately, medication served to control his seizures, for it was extremely difficult to find a conditioning approach to this highly complex evoking mechanism.

Medications may also play a significant but less obvious role in the complex types of reflex epilepsy. Here, medications may prevent the occurrence of major motor seizures without decreasing the incidence of minor seizures. This would appear to be true in reading epilepsy. Ten of the study patients with reading epilepsy had had major motor seizures while reading, but apparently none of them did after the introduction of antiepileptic medications. Moreover, it was not possible to evoke any major seizures in any of these patients in the laboratory situation, despite great amounts of reading.

The same situation with regard to major motor seizures occured in patients with musicogenic and in the case of voice-induced epilepsy (Case 10, Chapter 3). The latter patient had minor seizures characterized chiefly by aphasia with EEG discharges, particularly in the left temporal lobe. When her medications were discontinued for a very short period of time in order to complete the EEG studies, the presentation of the stimulus evoked an aphasic seizure followed by a generalized major motor seizure. This happened also in the first patient with musicogenic epilepsy when his medication was interrupted for the same purpose (detailed EEG study). These observations in reading epilepsy, voice-induced, and musicogenic epilepsy suggest that adequate doses of medications, particularly of hydantoinates and primidone, prevent the evoked minor seizures from progressing into major motor seizures in the patients with the complex types of reflex epilepsy.

While the hydantoinates and primidone seem to be the anti-convulsant medications of choice in the complex or secondary type of reflex epilepsy, studies in the laboratory suggest that nordiazepam is efficacious, at least for a time, in some of the patients with the simple or primary type of reflex epilepsy.

This medication was administered to photosensitive patients with resultant successful blocking of their dysrhythmia, thus obviating the need for conditioning treatment. One patient who was refractory to conditioning therapy (Case 35, Chapter 2) responded immediately to the administration of nordiazepam. He has a very occasional spontaneous major seizure but no longer has visually induced seizures or dysrhythmia.

One patient with auditory-induced epilepsy (Case 5, Chapter 3) also had complete control of his seizures upon the administration of nordiazepam. However, this was temporary, and after four weeks the effect gradually diminished. Thereafter, increasing dosages, even to the toxic point, did not affect the seizure frequency. It would seem then that in the simple or primary type of reflex epilepsy the benzodiapine therapy plays a significant role, although this may be a temporary effect.

Obviously, it would be much simpler to treat these patients with medications rather than with the various behavioral methods described herein. Most of the patients were referred because adequate dosages (with adequate therapeutic blood levels of the appropriate antiepileptic drugs) had not succeeded in bringing about seizure control.

Every patient admitted for these studies was maintained on the medication he or she was taking. Moreover, these medications were maintained at the same dosages during and after the conditioning process. However, the findings detailed in the following chapter cannot be attributed to these medications. It should also be noted that the seizures reported in these patients with reflex epilepsy were evoked under laboratory conditions despite the medications prescribed.

The therapeutic process, to test its efficacy, was also employed on occasion without the patient being on medication. For example, two photosensitive patients, Cases 1 and 14, Chapter 2, never received antiepileptic medications, and the conditioning process alone was successfully employed.

The behavioral methods of therapy in reflex epilepsy can therefore succeed either independent of medication or when medications have failed to control the clinical condition.

In summary, patients should be selected for behavioral therapies only when their seizures are definitely reflex in origin, when the seizures are severe enough to warrant therapy, and when they are uncontrolled by the usual antiepileptic medications. In addition, there must be adequate motivation, and progressive degenerative disease should preferably not be present.

CHAPTER 15

BEHAVIORAL THERAPY OF REFLEX
EPILEPSY: RESULTS

IN THIS CHAPTER are presented the results of applying the afore-mentioned treatment principles and methods to the study series of patients. In the preceding chapter, the criteria for case selection have been described and accordingly, certain patients were excluded from therapy. Since these criteria were developed during the course of the studies on behavioral therapy, some patients were included for therapy who, later and quite properly, would have been excluded. Nevertheless, these patients are listed as failures in treatment.

VISUALLY INDUCED EPILEPSY

Photosensitivity

Of the thirty-four patients with photosensitivity, thirteen were excluded from therapy. Table XVII presents the reasons for these exclusions as described in the preceding chapter. Four patients with infrequent seizures or who responded promptly to anticonvulsant medication were excluded from treatment in

TABLE XVII

PATIENTS WITH PHOTOSENSITIVITY EXCLUDED FROM
BEHAVIORAL THERAPY

Insufficient clinical seizures	2	(Cases 28 and 38)
Seizures controlled by medication	2	(Cases 18 and 23)
Poor cooperation	5	(Cases, 3, 6, 8, 12, and 24)
Too frequent spontaneous seizures	3	(Cases 19, 20, and 36)
Total	12	

Case numbers refer to Table II, in Chapter 2.

this laborious way. Five patients were excluded because of poor cooperation. They had varying degrees and combinations of severe retardation, marked hyperactivity, and inability of the patient and/or parents to cooperate in continuing the reinforcement process. The laboratory process could be carried out successfully using the monocular method, as in Case 7, or the differential light intensity, as in Case 3, but success in the laboratory is useless if reinforcement cannot be continued.

In three patients, the frequency of spontaneous dysrhythmia and seizures was so great that conditioning was not considered feasible.

Table XVIII presents a summary of the twenty-one patients

TABLE XVIII

BEHAVIORAL THERAPY IN PHOTOSENSITIVITY

A. Patients treated monocularly and using intermittent monocular reinforcement

Treated successfully	4
Unsuccessful	1
Total	5

B. Patients treated with DLI and using second-signal system for reinforcement

Treated successfully	9
Partial success	2
Unsuccessful	3
Unknown	2
Total	16

with photosensitivity who were treated with behavioral methods. Five patients were treated using the monocular method. Table XIX presents these patients and the medical data and results of the treatment.

All five patients were successfully treated in the laboratory using the monocular method. However, one patient (Case 7) would not continue the daily reinforcement stimulations when he left the hospital and is therefore considered a treatment failure. This patient appropriately should have been excluded from the study. Four patients maintained their conditioning after the successful laboratory process and continued their daily monocular reinforcements at home for periods ranging from one year (Case 17) to twenty-seven months (Case 14). The patients

TABLE XIX

Visually Induced Epilepsy
Monocular Therapy and Reinforcement

Case #	Sex	Age	Age of Onset	Seizure Type	Kinds of Visually Induced Epilepsy			Self-Stimulated	Results	Duration of Reinforcement
					Photic	Pattern	EC			
1	F	21	18	PM & MM	+	-	-	0	Seizure-free 6 yrs.	3 yrs.
7	M	10	8 mo.	PM & MM	+	-	-	0	Unsuccessful	None
13	F	13	12	PM	+	-	-	0	Seizure-free 5 yrs.	18 mos.
14	F	19	10	PM & MM	+	-	-	0	Seizure-free 7 yrs.	27 mos.
17	F	21	14	MM & PM	+	-	-	0	Seizure-free 5 yrs.	1 yr.

Case numbers refer to Table II in Chapter 2.

returned their portable stroboscopes and have remained seizure free for follow-up periods ranging from three years (Case 13) to seven years (Case 14). Two of these patients returned for follow-up study in the laboratory. Photic stimulation in one of these patients (Case 14) showed, only at maximum intensity, a photoconvulsive EEG evoked dysrhythmia but without clinical seizure. In the other patient (Case 13) only a photomyoclonic response was obtained at time of follow-up.

Table XX presents the results in sixteen patients treated with the differential light intensity technique and with reinforcement through the use of the specially designed second-signal glasses. Tables XVIII and XX present the data on these patients. The differential light intensity technique with reinforcement was successful in nine patients. These patients have remained free of visually induced seizues from three to eleven years after therapy was instituted. Four of the patients required a second laboratory session, about one year after the original treatment. Six of the nine patients returned their second-signal system glasses after periods of one to three years and have remained seizure free.

Three patients have continued to wear the glasses. Cases 9 and 10 are brothers. They state that when they remove their glasses in sunlight to clean them, they feel somewhat light-headed and are quite certain seizures would recur if they did not continue to wear them, even though they have had no seizures for eight years. One patient (Case 27) has likewise continued to wear her glasses for the past ten years.

In two cases, partial success was obtained. Both patients were treated successfully in the laboratory, returned home wearing the second-signal glasses, and were seizure free while wearing them. However, after a year one patient (Case 30) had some emotional problems, stopped wearing the glasses, and had a recurrence of seizures. A similar experience occurred in another patient (Case 22). He would wear his glasses only intermittently. Of course, the conditioning effect cannot be maintained under these conditions.

In three patients the treatment process was unsuccessful. In Case 35 who was both photosensitive and had eye-closure evoked

TABLE XX

Visually-Induced Epilepsy Treated With DLI and Second-Signal System

Case No.*	Sex	Age	Age of Onset	Seizure Type	Kinds of Visually Induced			Number of Therapy Sessions	Duration S.S.S.	Follow-up Period	Results
					Photic	Pattern	EC				
2	F	12	9	PM & MM	+	0	0	2	3 yrs.	11 yrs.	C
4	M	13	7	PM & MM	+	0	0	2	1 yr.	2 yrs.	C
5	M	22	6	PM	+	0	0	5	7 yrs.	7 yrs.	C
9	M	18	6	PM & MM	+	0	0	1	8 yrs.	8 yrs.	C
10	M	18	6	PM & MM	+	0	0	1	8 yrs.	8 yrs.	C
11	M	16	12	PM	+	0	0	1	—	Died	?
15	F	12	9	PM & MM	+	0	0	1	3 yrs.	5 yrs.	C
16	F	17	13	PM & MM	+	0	0	1	3 yrs.	4 yrs.	C
21	M	23	17	MM & Myoclonic	+	0	0	2	1 yr.	2 yrs.	U
22	M	18	13	Myoclonic	+	+	0	2	Inconsistent	3 yrs.	PC
26	F	16	2	PM & MM	+	+	0	1	Refused	2 yrs.	U
27	F	13	3	PM & MM	+	+	0	3	12 yrs.	10 yrs.	C
29	F	19	8	PM & MM	+	+	0	3	3 yrs.	3 yrs.	C
30	F	12	8	PM & MM	+	+	0	1	1 yr.	16 mos.	PC
31	F	13	1	PM & MM	+	+	0	1	Inconsistent	1 wk.	?
35	M	12		PM & MM	+	0	+	4	3 yrs.	3 yrs.	U

*refers to the same case histories
as examined in Table II.

Case numbers refer to Table II in Chap. 2.

C = Seizures controlled
PC = Seizures partially controlled
U = Unsuccessful
? = Unknown. Lost to follow-up

dysrhythmia, four prolonged attempts were made in the laboratory to achieve the conditioned effect. The differential light intensity technique was employed, and monocular presentations were coupled with this by patching one eye during the computer automated process. Also, prolonged sessions with eyes open and with eyes closed were tried. All were unsuccessful in achieving meaningful results.

The failure in this patient may have been due to the combination of photosensitivity and eye closure, or because this patient became aware of the significance of the automated ambient light changes and interpreted these as indications that the treatment process was not going well. Because of this experience, as noted before, the separate cubicle was designed in order to cut down on the effect of person to person contact.

In two patients with cerebellar myoclonus (Cases 21 and 26), therapy was unsuccessful. Case 26 also was very uncooperative during the laboratory phase of the treatment, so much so that the therapy required three instead of the usual two weeks. She resented wearing her glasses and, upon returning to her special school, destroyed the second-signal system glasses. This patient reinforces the primary criteria for exclusion of cases of poor cooperation and progressive disease processes.

The results of two cases are listed as unknown. Case 11 died of an unrelated cause, and the results are indeterminate. One patient (Case 31) could probably be considered a partial success. She previously persistently self-induced her seizures by finger waving. She learned that after the treatment process she could induce seizures by finger waving only when she did so in a manner to avoid stimulating the photoelectric cell. Thus she demonstrated the efficacy of the second-signal system.

Pattern Epilepsy

Six of the sixteen photosensitive patients also had pattern epilepsy. The laboratory phase of their treatment included the presentation of the patterns, usually in combination with the stroboscopic stimulation, and using the differential light intensity method. Success was obtained in two, partial success in two;

one patient represented a failure, and in one the results are tabulated as unknown.

This may suggest that a combination form of visually induced epilepsy is harder to treat than is a single form. The observations on the patient with photic and eye closure seizures would tend to corroborate this. However, the series is too small to draw a pessimistic conclusion regarding the therapeutic expectations when multiple forms of visually induced epilepsy are present.

Table XXI presents special treatment attempts. Included

TABLE XXI

OTHER THERAPEUTIC ATTEMPTS IN VISUALLY INDUCED EPILEPSY

Case	Sex	Age	Age at Onset	Kind of Visually Induced Epilepsy
25	F	11	6	Pattern epilepsy with some photosensitivity
32	F	9	6 mo.	Pattern only
37	F	19	18	Eye closure
39	M	5		Color/object-induced

are two additional cases of pattern epilepsy. The problem in Case 25 (Chapter 2) was predominantly pattern-evoked epilepsy. In the laboratory, she could be treated successfully with a combination of differential light intensity and altered focus of the patterns. The images of the patterns were prepared on a special cassette film for her with variations of illumination and focus, and the patient returned to her home. However, her family lacked the skills to maintain the cassette and movie projector in operation. Permanent success was not obtained.

Another patient (Case 32) was pattern sensitive only. Efforts at treatment were hampered here by severe retardation (I.Q. 39) and a very poor attention span. Numerous attempts were made to include the evoking patterns (horizontal and vertical lines) into pictures which might attract her attention. The focus and illumination would then be altered. Because of poor cooperation, however, it was impossible to achieve any significant results.

Eye Closure

The patient with eye closure dysrhythmia only (Case 37) was treated successfully in the laboratory, using the monocular method and also the differential light intensity technique, beginning the eye closure in darkness and gradually increasing the illumination level. For reinforcement, she was instructed to continue these methods at home. However, she also had psychiatric problems which necessitated her hospitalization in an appropriate institution, thus interrupting the therapeutic process.

Color/Object

The effect of avoidance conditioning in the patient with color/object-induced epilepsy (Case 39) has been discussed in Chapter 12. The administration of skin shocks dissuaded him from self-induction of seizures, but subsequent detailed psychometric evaluation showed no evidence of educability, and he was allowed to regress to his former state.

AUDITORY-EVOKED EPILEPSY

The simple form of auditory-evoked epilepsy (acousticomotor or startle epilepsy) can be readily treated in the laboratory by the stimulus alteration methods. The author and his colleagues have previously reported on the first two patients in this series.[1] When the first two patients were studied, the laboratory personnel were not aware of the importance of reinforcement or maintenance of the conditioning process after the laboratory treatments. For the third patient, an attempt was made at reinforcement therapy by devising an audiotape which the family could play several times a day over their home intercom system so as to present, daily, a sufficient number of stimulations. This patient remained seizure free. However, the family physician had changed the anticonvulsant medications, so it was not possible to establish whether the relief from seizures was the result of medication or of behavioral therapy.

Case 4 could be rendered free of seizures in the laboratory, and was given a tape to listen to at home. This was unsuccessful. Cases 3 and 4 were studied at the time of the first study patient with musicogenic epilepsy, hence the emphasis on the listening to tapes. The differences between simple and complex types of reflex epilepsy were not yet understood, hence the inappropriate application of reinforcement methods suitable in the complex type to the simple type.

However in reviewing the data on the second-signal system for photosensitivity, it became obvious that it was necessary to develop the second-signal system for the treatment of sound-induced seizures as described in Chapter 13. This system was employed in Cases 5 and 6, Chapter 3. Case 6, who was quite retarded, refused to wear the second-signal system apparatus after returning home. Case 5, however, after two weeks of treatment in the laboratory returned home. During the ensuing twelve months he had an occasional seizure not related to sound. The only sound-evoked seizures occurred when he had removed the second-signal system when preparing for bed or to shower. This occurred only twice. He was able to return to high school, graduate, and engage in full activities. Followup study in the laboratory demonstrated no seizures or dysrhythmia evoked by sound stimuli.

No behavioral therapeutic approach could be designed for the patients whose seizures were evoked by telephone bells or telephone transmission. Since the responses were impossible' to evoke in the laboratory, the evoking stimulus was never isolated. This was also true of the patient with seizures evoked by nonspecific voices.

The patient with seizures evoked by specific voices was successfully treated in the laboratory[2] and discharged from the hospital with her audio tapes, to which she listened twice a day. She has remained seizure free in the intervening nine years. Approximately three years ago, after five years of seizure freedom, her tape recorder fell into disrepair and she stopped listening to the tapes, but she has not developed seizures again despite adequate exposure to the voices of the announcers. It should be noted that during this time her anticonvulsant medications have been progressively decreased.

It would appear that after the passage of time, probably several years, the auditory reinforcement, like the second-signal system or the monocular reinforcement in photosensitivity, can be abandoned without the recurrence of seizures.

MUSICOGENIC EPILEPSY

Five patients with musicogenic epilepsy failed to respond to appropriate anticonvulsant medication and were accordingly treated with the behavioral techniques described. In the first patient, treatment was begun with a stimulus alteration technique as noted and was successful but too laborious, and for the remainder of the music to which he was sensitive, the threshold alteration technique was employed.[3] In the other four patients, no attempt was made to alter the stimulus, and the threshold alteration method was employed initially. All five patients were supplied with reinforcing tapes and advised to listen to them at least twice a day.[4]

Case 1, throughout the remainder of his life (ten years), was unable to have a seizure evoked by any of the tapes of music to which he had been treated in the laboratory or by any of the music which had been determined to be innocuous for him. He did, however, have a secondary gain in having seizures, since the occurrence of seizures made it possible for him not to seek gainful employment.

While in the hospital, he had a readily identifiable pseudo-seizure. On leaving the hospital, he listened faithfully to his reinforcing tapes and to the music that was delivered to him, without having seizures. He also listened avidly to all types of music. He did manage on occasion to find a musical number which would evoke a seizure. This happened for example when a particular singing star died, and during the Memorial Program on TV, the patient had a seizure evoked by the music. He went to the local library and obtained some fifty-seven different numbers sung by this particular star and listened to them consecutively without evoking a seizure! Thus he inadvertently extended still further his conditioning to music, and after that, he was no longer able to evoke seizures by means of this particular star's music. The patient subsequently died of pneumonia.

The second patient with musicogenic epilepsy had her seizures evoked by a restricted type of music—cowboy western music presented in relatively amateurish renditions. With this narrowly restricted range of evoking stimuli, the problem was simple. She was followed for five years after leaving the laboratory, continued to listen to her tapes, and was seizure free.

The third patient with musicogenic epilepsy has been able to attend church, go to the theatre, eat in restaurants with music, and to lead a complete life. For twenty years prior to treatment, she had avoided music. She has also returned to playing the piano. She has a very occasional seizure, usually when she has an infection or difficulty controlling her diabetes. These are not definitely linked to music, and certainly not to the kinds of music to which she had been conditioned.

The fourth patient had lost his job as a school teacher because of his musicogenic seizures. After the first conditioning session in the laboratory he did not faithfully carry out the maintenance therapy, and the seizures recurred. After the passage of six months, he returned to the laboratory for another conditioning session, using the same music, and now continues the maintenance therapy. He has been seizure free for two years and has returned to teaching.

The fifth patient is still in the process of achieving complete seizure control. The types of music comprising her evoking stimuli unfortunately include modern ballads, in which experimentation is continuing. She is free of seizures to the music to which she was conditioned but listens almost constantly to the radio. She occasionally has a seizure to some new number, one for which she has not been treated.

This patient also has a serious medical problem with renal artery occlusion and hypertension, with repeated surgical therapy becoming necessary for this condition. The medical problem, of course, takes precedence over the musicogenic epilepsy.

READING EPILEPSY

Of the eleven patients with reading epilepsies, only one could not benefit by the vigilance procedure (Case 5, Chapter 5). Case 3 was so uncooperative that it was not possble to determine the effectiveness of vigilance. In the other nine patients, this method was effective in the laboratory. It has not been successful, however, in permanently abolishing the seizures. This is probably because the signalling of the letters becomes almost a habit. The second patient noted when reading extensively (five hundred pages of text over a weekend) he had to change the letter he was signalling about every fifty pages. The Research Laboratory has yet to find a completely satisfactory behavioral method for treating these patents. It should be noted here, as previously described in Chapter 12, that the complete avoidance of reading in two patients was successful. Also, in one patient (Case 9, Chapter 5), after learning the results of the laboratory studies, partial avoidance was a successful method of treatment.

DECISION-MAKING EPILEPSY

As was noted before, the patient with decision-making epilepsy had his seizures controlled by medication. The study has at this time evolved no method for behavioral treatment of this form of reflex epilepsy.

SOMATOSENSORY-EVOKED EPILEPSY

The first patient with somatosensory-evoked epilepsy was studied many years before the conditioning process was even conceptualized. Postoperatively she has remained seizure free except for a generalized seizure four years ago when she was in a preeclamptic state.

The second patient, who also had the simple type of reflex epilepsy, was successfully conditioned in the laboratory. It was obvious that the conditioning needed reinforcement, thus the special switching device as described in Chapter 13 was designed and built. The patient, insisted, however, that the device be limited in size so she could wear very short skirts, and thus the reflexogenous zone could not be completely covered. The switching device on her leg could be activated only by a tapping. This would not happen frequently in her day-to-day environment, unlike the light changes which occur in nature and activate the special glasses for the photosensitive patients. She was instructed to self-stimulate at regular periods during the day so as to have adequate reinforcement.

Since she lived at a distance, two switching devices with sound-signal systems were made for her in case of malfunction of one of them. Four days after she left the hospital, she allowed her four-year-old child to dissemble one and let a radio amateur take the other one apart. This patient should not have been included for therapy because of her poor cooperation, which was obvious in the conditioning sessions as well as in the subsequent events just described. She was included for therapy because of the rarity of this particular form of reflex epilepsy. However, she does demonstrate that this simple type of somato-sensory reflex epilepsy can be conditioned in the laboratory but leaves the question open as to whether or not maintenance or recruitment therapy would be successful.

In the complex type of somatosensory-evoked epilepsy, further studies are necessary. Case 3, Chapter 7, developed a system of self-stimulation under controlled circumstances, namely in the morning before leaving for work. This resulted in a postictal refractory period which protected him for the remainder of the day. Attempts to graduate the evoking stimulus were tried in the hope of evoking a refractory period without the preceding clinical seizure. This, however, was not feasible. In Case 4, Chapter 7, because of the frequent spontaneous seizures and because anticonvulsant medications achieved reasonable success no behavioral method was designed.

SEIZURES EVOKED BY MOVEMENT

In the patient with seizures evoked by movement, because of limited laboratory time during the school year and adequate medications, behavioral methods were not undertaken As noted before, the proper use of antiepileptic medications controlled her seizures.

If medications had failed to control the seizures, the patient was to return in the summer vacation for an attempt at behavioral therapy. It is quite possible that suggestion might have alleviated her seizures, since the seizures could be evoked by suggestion.

EPILEPSY RELATED TO EATING

The first patient in the study series was so uncooperative that she could not be studied carefully, much less be involved in a course of behavioral therapy.

In the second patient with seizures evoked by eating, the evoking stimulus could not be defined more sharply. Since this type of reflex epilepsy, like reading epilepsy, is to some extent under the control of the patient, it seemed reasonable to try the vigilance technique. This was successful in the laboratory, and she was able to eat her meals without seizures when she indicated the onset of swallowing. However, the vigilance technique could not be extended to involuntary swallowing. She no longer had seizures associated with her meals, and after about one year discontinued the vigilance method. The seizures which occur now are only those occurring at times other than at meals.

The foregoing observations show that it is possible, by employing the appropriate behavioral techniques, to alter the clinical course of reflex epilepsy.

The question might be raised of coincidence of the cessation of seizures and the introduction of the treatments. However, these long term studies inevitably allowed some control observations.

CONTROL OBSERVATIONS ON EFFICACY OF BEHAVIORAL TREATMENT

The coincidental disappearance of seizures and dysrhythmia is extremely unlikely in view of the rather large number of patients involved, for example thirteen of the twenty-one patients with photosensitive epilepsy. Moreover, a conditioning effect was definitely shown in Case 1 Chapter 2 for the particular frequencies employed in the monocular treatment process, while other frequencies both above and below those still evoked seizures.

Case 3 (Chapter 2), for whom the second-signal system glasses were first designed, served as an admirable control. Weekly sessions with the differential light intensity method did not produce a lasting beneficial effect. When the second-signal system glasses were ready, she had a two-week session in the laboratory while wearing glasses.

Upon returning home, she remained seizure free except when, under unusual circumstances, she had two seizures. Both occured when she was not wearing her glasses. The first was while shampooing her hair, when she inadvertently passed her fingers before her eyes while looking up at the light. The second seizure occurred while using an electric cake mixer. The reflected light from the beaters kept her glasses clicking. She removed the glasses and promptly had a seizure. She then learned to avoid these types of intermittent visual stimulations while not wearing her glasses.

She continued seizure free for eighteen months. Her glasses needed repair, so she put them aside. After six months, the seizures returned. The glasses were repaired and she was again reconditioned in the laboratory, wearing her glasses, and became seizure free. After an additional twelve months, she again attempted her activities without the glasses, had no seizures, returned them to the laboratory, and has remained seizure free.

A control evaluation was also possible in the patient with voice-induced epilepsy (Case 10, Chapter 3). In November, 1967, the patient received behavioral or conditioning therapy for the three known voices which had evoked her seizures. These were the voices of three radio announcers. Once she had been conditioned in the laboratory to these voices, she returned home, listened to the prepared tapes two or more times per day, and listened to these announcers on their radio programs. She also called them on the telephone occasionally (without evoking seizures) to thank them for their cooperation. She was seizure free until mid-February, 1968.

While listening to the radio, she again had some seizures, decided the conditioning was a failure, and discontinued the reinforcement. Two weeks later she learned that there was a new announcer on her local station, and she and her husband realized that it was his voice that had evoked the seizures.

She returned to the conditioning laboratory and, upon listening to her tapes of the original three voices, seizures and dysrhythmia occurred. She had lost her conditioning by not listening daily to the tapes! The conditioning was reinstituted by the replaying of the tapes as before. The fourth announcer was contacted, and he also prepared a tape. This evoked a seizure in the laboratory, and she was conditioned to this voice as well. This tape then was added to her tapes for daily listening. No further seizures occurred in the subsequent eight years.

This sequence of events presents the control observation on the use of the tape of the original voices. Premature cessation of daily reinforcement allowed the conditioning to wear off.

A similar observation was deliberately made on our first patient with musicogenic epilepsy. He was allowed to return home for a period of three weeks during the early phase of his treatment process. At that time, laboratory testing had discovered six musical numbers which had evoked seizures. He had been treated for these, using the stimulus alteration method. Five of these numbers, but not the sixth number, were placed on his reinforcement tape. When he returned to the laboratory, the six numbers were presented. No seizures or dysrhythmia occurred with the five numbers to which he had listened twice daily while at home. The sixth number, to which he had not been exposed for reinforcement, evoked a seizure as soon as it was played.

As previously noted, the fourth patient with musicogenic epilepsy stopped listening to his tapes and had a recurrence of seizures; a second session in the laboratory was necessitated.

These observations in both the simple type (photosensitivity) and the complex types (voice-induced and musicogenic) of reflex epilepsy confirm the efficacy of the conditioning and the reinforcement or maintenance of the therapeutic process, and remove the possibility of chance spontaneous disappearance of seizures.

EXTENSION OF THERAPY IN THE HOME ENVIRONMENT

It was noted that one of the patients with musicogenic epilepsy (Case 1), in a deliberate attempt to induce seizures with particular music, had succeeded in furthering his conditioning by repeated applications of the stimulus. This suggested the possibility that enlightened patients, and especially enlightened families, can extend the conditioning therapy when necessary.

In Case 3 (Chapter 4) of musicogenic epilepsy, when she returned home, her sister tape recorded all the music to which they listened over the radio or TV. In that way, if a seizure occurred to a particular number, she was ready to replay the number over and over, and thus be able to add it to the music which no longer evoked seizures. Her sister also added such numbers to the "master tape" to which the patient listened daily.

This family's cooperation is not peculiar to the complex types of reflex epilepsy. In the visually induced group, Case 27 (Chapter 2), was both photic and pattern sensitive, was carefully conditioned and sent home with reinforcement, employing the special glasses and also the daily presentation of the offending patterns while hand waving to induce auditory clicks from her special glasses. About one year later, the author happened to be visiting her home in a distant part of the country. Her parents commented that she was doing very well except of late she had been having seizures on rising in the early morning. On inspecting her bedroom, it was obvious that the screen on the east window was newly replaced. Rather than returning her to the laboratory for conditioning of the screen effect, the simplest and best technique was to awaken the youngster before sunup, have her stand at the window looking through the screen and waving her hand for the induction of auditory clicks. The rising sun took the place of the laboratory rheostat. Her early morning seizures disappeared.

SPECIFICITY AND GENERALIZATION OF THE CONDITIONING EFFECT

The application of the behavioral techniques of stimulus alteration and threshold alteration has a conditioning effect and therefore there are factors of specificity and of generalization.

The evoking stimulus that is employed in either of these techniques becomes innocuous, thus showing a specificity. When the stroboscopic stimulations are presented at a given frequency, that frequency, after the treatment process, no longer evokes a dysrhythmia or seizure. The same is true of a startling sound, a particular voice, or a musical number. The specificity is shown for example in photosensitivity by the early observations in Case 1 (Chapter 2) whose photosensitive range extended from fifteen to thirty-five frequencies per second. After she was treated at twenty cycles per second, no seizures occurred upon repeated stimulation at frequencies from eighteen to twenty-two cycles per second. However, when she complained of having seizures at home when turning off the kitchen fan and watching the blades rotate in the sun, she was checked more carefully in the laboratory. She was insensitive to stimulations between eighteen and twenty-two cycles per second but still photosensitive between fifteen and eighteen, and twenty-two and thirty-five cycles per second. There is therefore a slight generalization of approximately five cycles per second.

Specificity is shown in the case of voice-induced epilepsy by the fact that the original three voices never evoked a seizure after completion of the conditioning process, whether heard taped or over the telephone, except when the patient interrupted the reinforcement.

Generalization occurs in both the simple and complex types. Some generalization is indicated in the above observations on photosensitivity, since not only the specific frequency that was altered failed to evoke seizures, but a narrow band of five cycles per second had also become innocuous. In acousticomotor epilepsy, conditioning to the sound of a particular bell or buzzer produces a generalization of the nonevoking effect to similar-sounding bells or buzzers.

Generalization is most obvious in the treatment of musicogenic epilepsy. For example, Case 3 Chapter 4 was well aware that any of the Strauss waltzes would evoke seizures, and she and her sister agreed that the "Blue Danbue Waltz" was the most likely to do so. The treatment process was begun with the "Emperor Waltz." Once the playing of this number did not evoke seizures or dysrhythmia all the Strauss Waltzes were presented to her in serial fashion, including several renditions of the "Blue Danube." No dysrhythmia and no seizures were evoked. The same generalization phenomenon was seen in the other musicogenic patients.

In the patient with voice-induced epilepsy, generalization of the effect also occurred. This patient had seizures under many conditions when people were talking. Initially it was difficult to identify the stimulus as a particular voice. Yet the conditioning based upon the identifiable voices—those of radio announcers—led to the alleviation of seizures induced by other voices.

In planning the treatment process for a given patient, it is necessary to take into consideration the processes of generalization and of specificity. Generalization can be used to cover a number of very similar evoking stimuli, but it is necessary, in view of the specificity and in order to achieve the ultimate goal of seizure freedom, to search for and cover all possible contingencies.

In the patients with musicogenic epilepsy, this can be difficult if the evoking stimuli lie in music with which experimentation is being done at the present time. The third patient with musicogenic epilepsy presented a relatively simple problem for there are now no explorations in music forms similar to Tschaikovsky Ballets or Strauss Waltzes. However, the fifth patient with musicogenic epilepsy was affected by modern popular ballad music, a type of music undergoing extension and modification.

NEUROPHYSIOLOGIC EFFECTS OF
BEHAVIORAL THERAPY

There are specific neurophysiologic effects of the conditioning process. These consist of alterations of the evoked dysrhythmia and of the GSR changes when they occur.

During the course of the conditioning process, the dysrhythmia, whether primarily generalized or primarily focal in onset, is altered. It was noted in treating photosensitivity that after the differential light intensity conditioning technique is in operation for several days, changes in computer sensitivity levels need to be made. This is because the evoked dysrhythmia is then of a lower voltage and is not manifested to the computer soon enough. These changes are barely perceptible upon examining the paper records. The illustrations from the computer writeouts (Figs. 71, 72), however, show this. These writeouts were obtained from the computers in the Cybernetics Laboratory of the University of Wisconsin at the time of the pilot studies on computer automation.

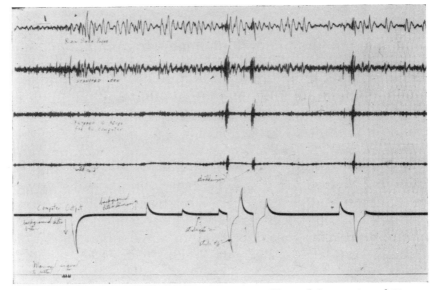

Figure 71.   Computer automation write-out. (From laboratories of Doctor K. U. Smith.) Four upper channels are EEGs as recorded by telephone transmission in Doctor Smith's laboratory. Fifth channel shows stimulus presentation and ambient light control. Upward deflections in fifth channel indicate decreasing steps in ambient room light. Evoked dysrhythmia triggered computer cessation of stroboscopic stimulation and produced increases in ambient room light (downward deflections of baseline). Note abrupt onset and magnitude of dysrhythmia. No clinical seizure.

Alteration of the evoked dysrhythmia also occurs in the complex type of reflex epilepsy. This is indicated by the observations in reading epilepsy.[5] Often the evoked dysrhythmia in reading epilepsy has the appearance of a bilateral or generalized dysrhythmia. However, when stimulus alteration conditioning is employed for treatment, a gradual alteration occurs in the evoked dysrhythmia. Case 1, Chapter 5 was treated first with a stimulus modification technique. He silently read the same material over and over. Of course, no dysrhythmia occurred since he had no seizures when reading silently. Such reading was innocuous. He then read aloud the same material until a dysrhythmia and/or a seizure occurred. At this point, he was returned to the memorized material for repeated silent readings. It was found that he could read for longer periods of time

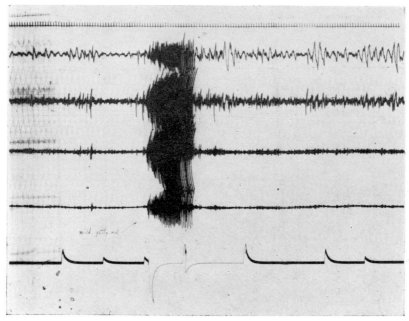

Figure 72. Same as preceding figure, but after ten hours of conditioning therapy. Onset of dysrhythmia is of lower magnitude and builds up rapidly into a full-blown seizure discharge. This indicates a therapeutically induced alteration of the evoked seizure responses.

without seizures after each session of reading silently. This method, however, was quite laborious for effective treatment. Nevertheless, it demonstrated that stimulus alteration conditioning affected the dysrhythmia (Fig. 73). The abnormal discharge became restricted to one anterior temporal lead, lost its sharpness, and decreased in amplitude. The slight sharp wave in the last tracing might be questioned as to its significance, but the patient was subjectively aware of a seizure and signalled it when it occurred in the record.

A similar but less dramatic alteration by conditioning of the evoked potential occurred in musicogenic epilepsy (Fig. 74). In Case 1, while he was being treated by the stimulus alteration method, a decrease in the evoked spiking discharges occurred, but the decrease was not as dramatic as in the case of reading epilepsy. However, when the threshold alteration method is

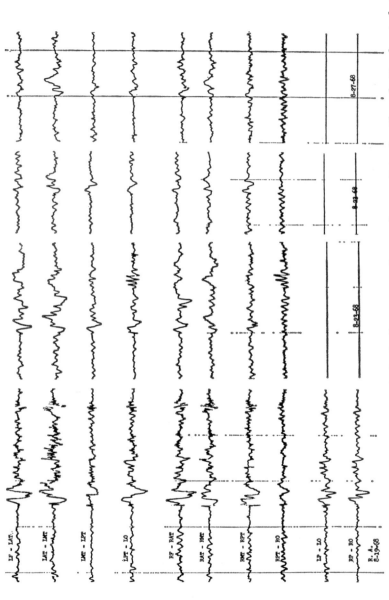

Figure 73. Neurophysiologic change in evoked dysrhythmia in reading epilepsy. Case 1. Altered stimulus technique of modifying evoked seizures. Four consecutive evoked dysrhythmias during conditioning process. Note decrease in sharpness of evoked spike from left anterior temporal region and associated decrease in transmission of discharge to other cortical areas. (Reprinted from *Neurology* © 1969 by The New York Times Media Company, Inc.

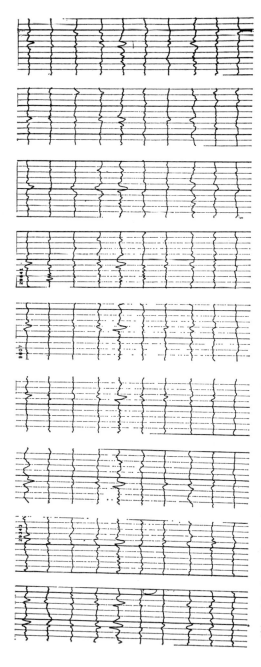

Figure 74. Musicogenic epilepsy. Case 1. Stimulus alteration type of conditioning therapy. Note decrease in left temporal spiking discharge (fifth channel), and decrease of spread to other areas. Gain constant.

READING EPILEPSY: EFFECT OF CONDITIONING ON EVOKED GSR RESPONSE

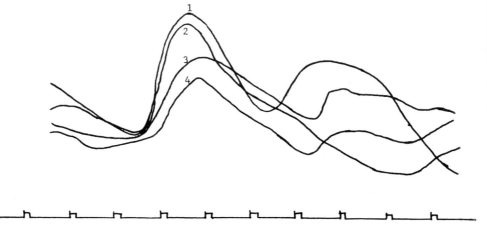

Figure 75.   Reading epilepsy. Case 1. Stimulus alteration type of conditioning. These GSR responses occurred with the evoked dysrhythmias shown in Figure 73. Note decrease in GSR changes correlating with similar changes in evoked cortical dysrhythmias. (Reprinted from *Neurology* © 1969 by The New York Times Media Company, Inc.

employed for conditioning and evokes a seizure, this gradual decline in the evoked dysrhythmia cannot be seen.

It has been noted that GSR changes occur in musicogenic and in reading epilepsy. As yet, a systematic survey has not been made of the autonomic responses in all forms of reflex epilepsy. The GSR changes are not related to awareness by the patient of the imminence of a seizure.

When the evoked cortical potential is altered by conditioning, so is the GSR change. This is demonstrated in Figure 75, which shows the GSR changes in the patient with reading epilepsy. These occurred with the dysrhythmia, as shown in Figure 73, and it is obvious that the strength of the GSR alteration was decreased as the evoked potential was ameliorated.[5]

The neurophysiological alterations induced by conditioning then indicate that the abnormal evoked potential is altered at the site of evocation and that the spread of the discharge is inhibited to other cortical areas as well as to subcortical structures. This latter is based on the supposition that hypothalamic structures are involved in the GSR changes.

In summary, the application of the appropriate behavioral method in a patient with well-defined reflex epilepsy and proper motivation results in improvement in the clinical condition, with underlying neurophysiological changes.

In embarking on the therapeutic process, and particularly when employing stimulus alteration methods, one must be constantly aware that it is possible to worsen the condition of a patient. The careless patching of the vision of one eye can readily eliminate monocular insensitivity. Beginning stimulations at the upper or lower edge of the photosensitive range and carrying them slowly outside the range can increase the range of sensitivity. Failure to appreciate a "hang up" in the computer automation procedure, and not introducing other variables such as monocular stimulation into the differential light technique at that point, may make the photosensitivity worse. Perhaps these possible worsening effects are limited to the simple type of reflex epilepsy, but one should be constantly aware of the delicate effect of a conditioning process upon the human central nervous system, especially upon a nervous system which, by virtue of having seizures, has indicated the presence of an instability.

REFERENCES

1. Booker, H. E., Forster, F. M., and Klove, H.: Extinction factors in startle (acoustico-motor) seizures. *Neurology, 15*:1095, 1965.
2. Forster, F. M., Hansotia, P., Cleeland, C. S., and Ludwig, A.: A case of voice induced epilepsy treated by conditioning. *Neurology, 19*:325, 1969.
3. Forster, F. M., Klove, H., Peterson, W. G., and Bengzon, A. R. A.: *Proc 8th Internat Cong Neurol, 4*:269, 1965.
4. Forster, F. M.: Human studies of epileptic seizures induced by sound and their conditioned extinction. In Welch, B. L. and Welch, A. S. (Eds.): *Physiological Effects of Noise.* New York, Plenum Pr., 1970.
5. Forster, F. M., Paulsen, W. A., and Baughman, F. A.: Clinical therapeutic conditioning in reading epilepsy. *Neurology, 19*:717, 1969.

CHAPTER 16

REFLEX EPILEPSY AND
CONDITIONAL REFLEXES

T HE POSSIBILITY THAT sensory-evoked epilepsy in animals and humans might be a manifestation of conditional reflexes has often been considered. The volume edited by Servit[1] considered the problem in detail, with particular emphasis on audiogenic seizures in animals. Critchley[2] was the first to consider that musicogenic epilepsy in the human might represent a conditional reflex but, after careful consideration, discarded the possibility. Shaw and Hill[3] again raised the possibility.

Exposure in 1958 to the work of Soviet colleagues evoked in the author the interest which has lead to this volume. The possibility seemed very likely that the reflex epilepsies could be conditional reflexes. It is interesting to note that various authors who have considered this possibility have done so in respect to the complex types of reflex epilepsy, for example musicogenic. This is probably because the evoking stimulus deals with mentation or higher cognitive functions.

In a previous communication in 1969,[4] the author dealt at length with the possibilities of conditional reflexes playing an etiological effect in reflex epilepsy, citing laboratory data in both experimental animals and in patients with reflex epilepsy. The possibility that a conditional reflex might play a role in the production of sensory-evoked epilepsy immediately allows the deduction that a behavioral type of therapy might be applicable. The author and his colleagues did not wish to begin the studies on patients but preferred rather to begin with animals in order to be in a better position to understand the process and also to avoid the possibility of harming the patients.

Accordingly, in 1959, a series of animal studies were begun, using implanted electrodes in cats with intact brains, and in 1963, the results of conditioning studies in animal preparations were presented.[5] The unconditioned stimulus (electrical stimulation to the motor cortex of one hemisphere) produced focal motor seizures on the opposite side of the body. The conditioning stimulus (sound or intermittent light) was administered for a four-second interval alone and then continued through a two-second period coupled with the unconditioned stimulus (US). After a series of trials, usually not fewer than twenty-five nor more than fifty, the animals developed behavioral and EEG changes upon presentation of the conditioning stimulus (CS).

The behavioral responses consisted of changes in posture preparatory to the onset of the focal seizures [unconditional reflex (UR)]. The exact nature of the preparatory response depended on the part of the body involved in the focal seizure and the personality of the cat. If the cat was docile, it tended to crouch, pull in its extremities, wrap its tail about itself and wait patiently. More aggressive cats would rise up on all fours and stand with their legs in a fixed position (Figs. 76A & 76B). If the hind leg was involved in the seizure, the animals also tended to stand. Failure to present the US after conditioning resulted in surprise, and the animal would turn its head to look at the member of the body ordinarily involved in the focal seizure.

The EEG changes consisted of augmentation and generalization of the primary cortical-evoked potential—e.g. the auditory-evoked spike occurring with the presentation of a sound (CS) at first appeared only in acoustic cortex but, as the conditioning process proceeded, the evoked potential was of higher amplitude and was evident over all areas of cortex, even on bipolar recordings from the motor cortex (Figs. 77A, 77B & 77C). This generalization of the evoked potential was followed by desynchronization and flattening of the brain waves from all areas until cessation of the conditioning stimulus. In cats with intact cerebral cortex, no seizure could be elicited by CS alone. Both behavioral and EEG changes induced by conditioning could be removed by extinction, i.e. by repeated presentation of the conditioning stimulus without reinforcement.

From these studies it was concluded that, while it is possible

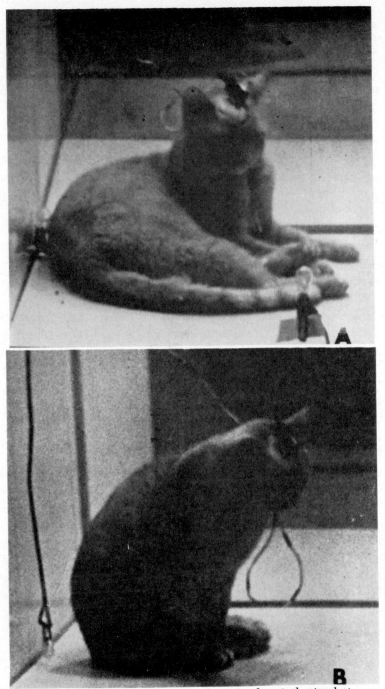

Figure 76. Cat 8. CS; sound (buzzer). US; electrical stimulation to left motor cortex with resulting (UR) focal seizure right upper extremity. After fifteen conditioning trials, on test trial, animal in resting state (Fig. 76A), upon presentation of CS, assumes the upright, alerted, clinical state (76B).

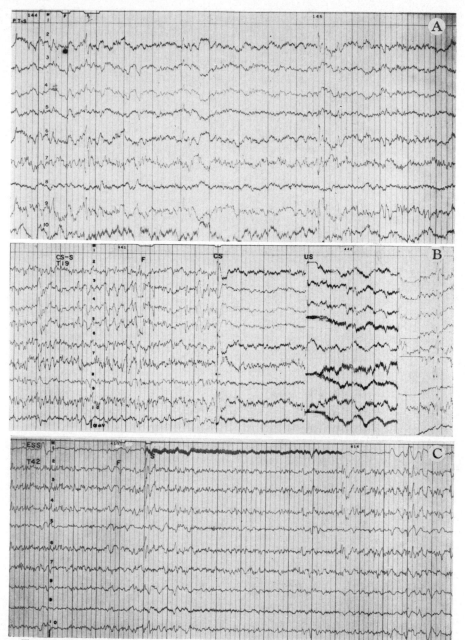

Figure 77. EEG tracings during conditioning studies in experimental epilepsy. A. Recording of first presentation of CS (sound). B. Recording of the 19th presentation of CS (sound) coupled with US (electrical stimulation of motor cortex). There is generalization of the cortical potentials evoked by the sound stimulus, followed by desynchronization of electrical activity for four seconds. Sixty-cycle artifact occurs to some extent during presentation of CS and in marked degree during the period of presentation of the US. C. Recording during the forty-second extinction

by conditioning to produce behavioral and EEG changes, it was not possible to evoke seizures as a conditional reflex (CR) in cats with intact brains.

Studies were then undertaken to render the brain epilepto-genic and to repeat these experiments. Induction of the destructive and epileptogenic lesion at the time of the original surgery for electrode implantation would interfere with the conditioning process. Likewise, a second anesthesia and surgical procedure after the conditioning had been established would destroy or alter the conditioning. To eliminate the need for a second operative procedure, a sterile plastic tube was inserted through the plastic cap when the electrodes were imbedded. The tube's open end was in contact with the dura, and the exterior end was sealed. Once conditioning had been well established, the exterior end of the tube was opened and epileptogenic material injected directly into the cortex.

In the early studies, after the animals had become conditioned, an acutely epileptogenic agent (Metrazol®, penicillin, picrotoxin, or strychnine) was injected intracortically and the conditioning stimulus gven. While it appeared that the conditioning stimulus evoked the appropriate seizure, the results were not conclusive because of the acute epileptogenic activity present. Moreover, the epileptogenic drug often produced a major convulsion which obliterated the conditioning already established.

Attempts were then made to produce a more chronic epileptogenic lesion. Implantations of lead and applications of dry ice were made through the plastic tube. These, however, led to a

---

trial (presentation of CS without presentation of US). The sound-evoked potential is no longer generalized and desynchronization has disappeared. Tope line ("M") is incident marker. "F" indicates starting of camera to film experiment; "CS," presentation of CS (sound); "US," presentation of US (electrical stimulation of the motor cortex). Electrical activity is recorded as folows: 1. paired electrodes over left motor cortex; 2. left motor to left anterior suprasylvian; 3. left anterior suprasylvian to left midectosylvian; 4. left midectosylvian to left midsuprasylvian; 5. left mid-suprasylvian to left postsuprasylvian; 6. right midectosylvian to right post-suprasylvian; 7. right postsuprasylvian to right posterior sylvian; 8. right posterior sylvian to right coronal; 9. right coronal to left motor cortex; 10. right posterior sylvian to right suprasylvian. (Reprinted from *Arch Neurol,* 9:188, 1963).

relatively small number of "takes." They were fraught with problems as to the time required for conditioning and for "ripening" of the lesion, and the uncertainty of developing an epileptogenic "take."

Subacute lesions were then induced. After the conditioning had been established, tetanus toxin was injected into the cortex. This procedure required twenty-four to forty-eight hours to produce an epileptogenic lesion. Evaluation of the effect of the CS was made before the epileptogenic lesion was sufficiently severe to lead to generalized convulsions, for these, of course, destroyed the conditioning. The tetanus toxin is in itself lethal, and mortality in these studies was high.

Table XXII presents the results of studies of nine cats with epileptogtnic lesions due to tetanus toxin. In each of the first four cats, the epileptogenic lesion was made in the primary cortical analyzer after conditioning was established. Three had lesions of the visual cortex; the conditioning stimulus was intermittent light. The other had a lesion of the acoustic cortex; the CS was sound. As the epileptogenic lesion "ripened," spontaneous spiking occurred prior to the development of clinical seizures. Presentation of the CS then resulted in a clinical seizure, similar in most respects to that evoked by the US. The clinical seizure was accompanied electroencephalographically by seizure dysrhythmia. The presentation of the neutral stimulus (sound or light) elicited no seizures. The results of this portion of the study, however, were open to question since, in these four cats, the primary cortical analyzer was the site of the lesion.

In the second group of five cats, the lesions of the cortex were not in the primary cortical analyzer. In a cat with a lesion of the visual cortex, and for which the CS was sound, the presentation of the CS, as soon as the cortex was epileptogenic, evoked a seizure, whereas the presentation of light did not. The second cat in this series had a lesion of the motor cortex, which might be considered the final common pathway regardless of the nature of the CS. For this cat, sound was the CS and, following the production of the epileptogenic lesion, it evoked a seizure, whereas light (the neutral stimulus) did not.

The last three cats in the second group were controls, studied

TABLE XXII

SENSORY EVOCATION OF SEIZURES BY CONDITIONING: CATS WITH EPILEPTOGENIC LESIONS

			Reaction			
			to CS		to NS	
Cat	Lesion*	CS	Clinical Response	EEG Response	Clinical Response	EEG Response
Lesion in the primary cortical analyzer						
17	V.C.	Light	Seizure	Seizure	0	0
25	V.C.	Light	Seizure	Seizure	0	0
19	A.C.	Sound	Seizure	Seizure	0	0
37	V.C.	Light	Seizure	Seizure	0	0
Lesion in the cortex, but not in the primary cortical analyzer						
21	V.C.	Sound	Seizure	Seizure	0	0
28	M.C.	Sound	Seizure	Seizure	0	0
Control US, no CS						
24	A.C.	—	—	—	0	0 L/S
23	V.C.	—	—	—	0	0 L/S
26	A.C.	—	—	—	0	0 L/S

* V.C. = visual cortex; A.C. = acoustic cortex; M.C. = motor cortex; L/S = light and sound. From Forster, F. M.: Conditioning in sensory evoked seizures. *Conditional Reflex, 1*:224, 1966.

at the same early stage of tetanus toxin-induced epilepsy. One had been subjected to an equivalent number of unconditioned stimuli — electrical stimulation producing the focal motor seizures — in other experiments. This cat had a lesion of the acoustic cortex and had not been conditioned. Neither light nor sound evoked seizures. The other two controls had received neither CS nor US, and no seizures were triggered by light or sound in the same early stage of epileptogenicity.

These experiments indicate that, by conditioning, it is possible to produce sensory-evoked seizures in animals as a CR. However, the seizures as a CR are difficult to acquire. They require an epileptogenic lesion plus repeated presentation of the conditioning stimuli coupled with an unconditioned stimulus.

A significant observation during these studies was that when inadvertent generalized convulsions were induced by the US, or by acute epileptogenic drug applications, the conditioning was obliterated and had to be reestablished. This was first noted in one cat by the accidental administration of a greater stimulus than necessary to evoke a focal seizure. To be certain that this was not an incidental finding, it was repeated in three more animals after they had attained their conditioning. Each time it was noted that after generalized seizures, conditioning was lost. This was true in both the first series of cats with normal intact brains and in the series of cats with the epileptogenic lesions.

CLINICAL AUGMENTATION AND INDUCTION OF REFLEX EPILEPSY BY CONDITIONING

As noted before, reflex epilepsy in patients can be made worse by errors in either the method of study or in the treatment process. In Chapter 2 it was noted that in determining the range of photosensitivity, the investigator must approach the suspected zone from the safest limits (single flash and flicker fusion). The converse leads to an increase in the range of photosensitivity. Likewise, in Chapter 12, the inadvertent production of monocular sensitivity occurred when there were errors in therapeutic technique. These are considered examples of conditioning effects achieved by stimulus alteration.

When these effects were first noted, the hypothesis that conditioning could make the patient more sensitive by altering the intensity of the stimulus was tested. In a patient, the minimum ambient light level at which photosensitivity could be evoked was determined. Following this, the room was completely darkened, and repeated bursts of dysrhythmia were induced by photic stimulation while the ambient light levels were slowly increased. The dysrhythmias could then be evoked at much higher levels of ambient illumination (see Fig. 78), thus demonstrating a conditioning effect making the patient more sensitive. The usual therapeutic procedure was then employed to remove the induced increment of photosensitivity.

The latter observations of stimulus intensity are of considerable importance in the treatment of patients using the differential light intensity method.

In some patients, when lowering of the ambient light by a single logarithmic step has allowed stroboscopic stimuli to evoke a dysrhythmia, raising the light by one logarithmic step to that last innocuous stage and restimulating with the stroboscope will evoke a seizure. By repeating at progressively higher single steps, this can be carried up to the point of maximum ambient light (600 footcandles). This "carrying up" phenomenon can be avoided when a noxious level of ambient light has occurred by increasing the room light by two or more logarithmic steps.

The most convincing indication that conditioning can play a role in developing such a clinical seizure is found in the study of a patient with startle epilepsy.[6] Photic stimulation evoked neither clinical nor EEG changes. The sound stimulus and the sound-evoked seizures were used as the US and UR and stroboscopic stimulation as the CS. Four seconds of stroboscopic stimulation (CS) followed by the startling noise (US) were presented to the patient. After fifty trials, stroboscopic stimulation alone was sufficient to induce the seizure discharge (Figs. 79A, 79B & 79C). Repeated presentation of the CS without reinforcement of the US led to extinction.

These experimental and clinical results indicate that it is possible for a conditioning process to play a role in the evolution and augmentation of sensory-evoked epilepsy.

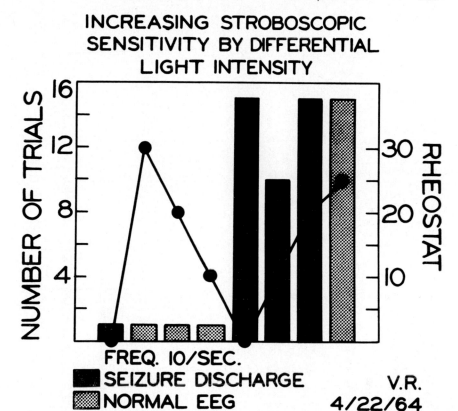

Figure 78. Conditioning effect in increasing photosensitivity. Ambient light levels are indicated by rheostat readings on right of graph. Patient was photosensitive in darkened room (ambient light turned off) but not at rheostat levels of 10 (approximately 50 foot candle light intensity). After repeated stimulations in dark, photosensitivity was present at much higher ambient room light levels. Repeated stimulation again decreased patient's sensitivity. Reprinted from *Arch Neurol, 11*:603, 1964.

WHY REFLEX EPILEPSY IS NOT A CONDITIONAL REFLEX

Although sensory-evoked seizures can be induced in animals by conditioning, and naturally occurring reflex epilepsy can be made worse or even transferred to a different category of reflex epilepsy by conditioning, it is unlikely that naturally occurring reflex epilepsy is a CR.

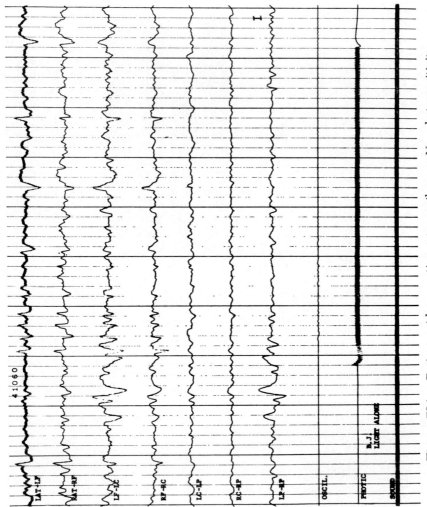

Figure 79A.   Patient with acousticomotor epilepsy.   No photosensitivity.
No EEG changes with photic stimulation.

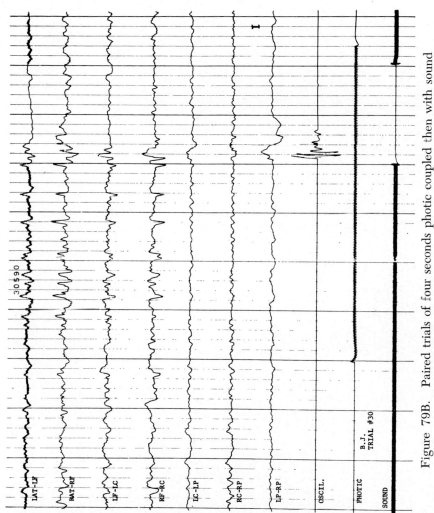

Figure 79B. Paired trials of four seconds photic coupled then with sound stimulation. Break in bottom channel, marked "sound," indicates administration of sound stimulus. Myoclonic seizure occurs as indicated by oscillometer attached to arm of patient.

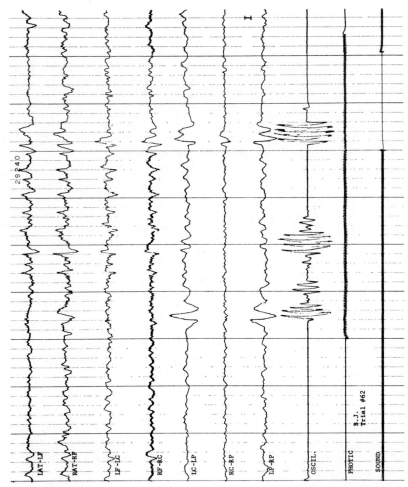

Figure 79C.   After sixty trials, photic stimulation alone evokes myoclonic seizure. Reprinted from *Neurology* ©1965 by The New York Times Medica Company, Inc.

It is true that light or sound stimuli can, by a conditioning process in cats with epileptogenic cortex, evoke a seizure as a conditional reflex. This reaction, however, is extremely difficult to accomplish and to maintain. The difficulty in itself casts some doubt on the possibility that reflex epilepsy is a conditional reflex.

Moreover, as was noted in the animal experiments, the accidental or purposeful induction of a major motor seizure obliterated the conditioning. Conditioning trials had to be reinstituted in order to reestablish the reflex. In the previous chapters, the high incidence of major motor seizures in patients with various forms of reflex epilepsy is quite obvious. Twenty-nine of the patients with visually induced epilepsy and all of the patients with musicogenic epilepsy had had major motor seizures. Nine and possibly ten of the patients with reading epilepsy had had convulsions in response to reading. Nevertheless, the patients had minor seizures evoked by the appropriate stimuli.

When medications were reduced in the patient with voice-induced epilepsy, presentation of the specific voices induced major motor convulsions; when medications were reinstituted, the presentation of the voices induced focal seizures. In a patient with musicogenic epilepsy (Case 1, Chapter 4), reduction of medication on three occasions led to the evocation of major motor seizures by the music. After reinstitution of full doses of medication, presentations of music evoked psychomotor seizures. Therefore, the reflex-evoked focal epilepsy was in no way ameliorated in either patient by the sensory-evoked major motor seizures. The abolitional effect of major motor convulsions on conditional reflexes was previously noted by Peters.[7] The persistence of focal-evoked seizures after the occurrence of major motor seizures also suggests that the reflex epilepsies are not conditional reflex in nature.

The following factor is of great importance to the point of view that reflex epilepsy is not a conditional reflex. If reflex epilepsy were a CR, it would be necessary to postulate a precise application of the stimulus (CS) with spontaneously occurring seizures (UR) beyond the realm of possibility. This can be applied to any of the forms of reflex epilepsy. For example, if this possibility were applied to a patient with musicogenic epilepsy, it would mean that he would have had to hear the specific music or particular theme fifteen, twenty, or twenty-five times in a relatively short period of time during several months and have had a spontaneous seizure occurring each time. This type of music could not have been heard at any other time, nor could he have had any other spontaneous seizures. These mathematical odds are obviously remote.

The necessity for a maintenance or reinforcement of the conditioning therapy, whether attained by stimulus alteration or threshold alteration, is a further indication that the evoked seizures are not conditional reflexes. If they were, one would expect deconditioning to remove the seizure without the necessity of a continuing reinforcement.

Each of these arguments standing alone is not sufficient evidence to establish that naturally occurring reflex epilepsy is definitely not based upon a conditional reflex. However, the sum total of the arguments makes this premise a persuasive one.

REFERENCES

1. Servit, Z.: *Reflex Mechanisms in the Genesis of Epilepsy.* Amsterdam, London, New York, Elsevier, 1963.
2. Critchley, M.: Musicogenic epilepsy. *Brain, 13*:6061, 1937.
3. Shaw, D. and Hill, D.: A case of musicogenic epilepsy. *J Neurol Neurosurg Psychiat, 10*:107, 1947.
4. Forster, F. M.: Conditioning in sensory evoked seizures. *Cond Reflex, 1*:224, 1966.
5. Forster, F. M., Chun, R. W. M., and Forster, M. D.: Conditioned changes in focal epilepsy. I. In animals with intact central nervous system. *Arch Neurol, 9*:188, 1963.
6. Booker, H. E., Forster, F. M., and Klove, H.: Extinction factors in startle (acousticomotor) seizures. *Neurology, 15*:1095, 1965.
7. Peters, J. E.: A comparison of the effect of two different types of electro-convulsive treatment on conditional reflexes in dogs. In Gantt, W. H. (Ed.): *Physiological Basis of Psychiatry.* Springfield, Thomas, 1958, pp. 53-70.

AUTHOR INDEX

A

Agreda, J. M., 42
Aird, R. B., 68
Alajouanine, T., 119-120, 123
Allen, J., 135, 155
Allen, J. M., 68
American Neurological Association,
 156
Ames, F. R., 43
Anderman, K., 43
Andermann, F., 43
Araki, S., 171
Arfel-Capdevielle, 122

B

Bailey, A., 122
Baird, H. W., 43
Balestra, F., 122
Barrios del Risco, P., 90, 93
Baughman, F. A., 241, 287
Baughman, F. A., Jr., 122
Baxter, D., 122
Behrman, S., 8, 10
Bengzon, A .R. A., 122, 182, 241, 287
Bennett, D. R., 97, 116, 120, 122, 240
Bennett, Maxine, 158
Berger, Hans, 3, 10
Bert, J., 41
Bickford, R., 94, 122
Bickford, R. G., 13, 22, 30-31, 41-42,
 45, 54-55, 67-68, 94, 122
Bingel, A., 122, 133-134
Blumenthal, I., 122
Blumenthal, I. J., 182
Booker, H. E., 44, 68, 182, 240-241,
 287, 302
Brazier, M. B., 3, 10
Brown, E., 69, 92, 182
Burger, L. J., 171
Burke, E. C., 42

C

Campos, G. B., 41, 182
Celesia, G. C., 12, 41
Charany, J. A., 122
Chatrian, G. E., 31-32, 42
Chen, L. T., 103, 121-122
Ch'en, Han-Pai, 133-134
Ch'in, Chen, 133-134
Chocholova, L., 201, 240
Chrast, B., 93
Ch'u, Chic-Ping, 133-134
Chun, R. W. M., 41, 182, 302
Cleeland, C. S., 63, 68, 155, 226, 240,
 241, 287
Clement, C. P., 43
Cohen, N. M., 44, 68
Cobb, S., 13, 41, 120
Cohen, N. M., 44, 68
Copalakrishnan, P. N., 155
Corrici, J., 68
Critchley, M., 45, 49-51, 68-69, 92, 107,
 120, 122, 288, 302
Cvetko, B., 41

D

Daly, D. D., 30, 31, 34, 38, 41-42, 42-
 43, 45, 54-55, 67-68
Daly, R. F., 122
Daube, J., 4, 10
Davidson, J. R., 43
Davidson, S., 42
Dongier, F. L., 43
Doose, H., 42
Doudoumopoulis, A. N., 9, 11
Dunn, A., 122
Dunn, A. T., 182
Dunsmore, J., 135, 154

303

SUBJECT INDEX

A

Abnormal discharges from brain, 3
Absence (*See* Petit mal)
Acousticomotor epilepsy, 44, 175, 258
   (*See also* Auditory-evoked
    epilepsy)
   behavioral therapy, 219-224
   cortical kind, 49
   intensity of stimulus, 87
   monaural stimulation, 87
   second-signal system device for,
    252-253
   subcortical kind, 49
   sudden unexpected nonspecific noise
    evoking, 45-49
Acousticomotor reflexes in children, 45
Adrenocorticotropic hormone (ACTH)
   therapy, 193
Adversive seizures, 45
   progressing to a major motor, 45
Age as factor, 28, 32, 74, 103
Alcohol as factor, 76, 125, 193
Alobar prosencephaly, 181
Alzheimer's disease, 29
Amnesia, 76, 99, 101-102, 132, 187
Amnestic aphasia, 64
Amphetamines, 47, 193, 198
Anectine, 49, 181
Aneurysm, 194
Anticonvulsant medication, 55, 70,
   72-73, 91, 139, 164, 190, 237,
   259-263, 272, 274-275 (*See also*
   specific types)
Antiepileptic medication (*See*
   Anticonvulsant medication *or*
   specific types)
Anxiety, 130, 133
Anxiety neuroses, 200

Aphasic and major motor seizures
   evoked by nonstartling and specific
   voices, 60-67
Aphasic seizures, 45, 83, 121, 176, 260
Apraxia, 161, 163
Arthrogryposis multiplex congenita,
   156
Astrocytoma, 59
Ataxia, 192, 194
Atypical spike and wave dysrhythmia,
   3, 13
Audiovisual monitoring with split-
   screen technique, 7
Auditory-evoked epilepsy, 8-9 (Table),
   44-68, 175, 179-180
   acousticomotor epilepsy evoked by
    sudden unexpected nonspecific
    noises, 45-49 (*See also*
    Acousticomotor epilepsy)
   aphasic and major motor seizures
    evoked by nonstartling and
    specific voices, 60-67
   behavioral therapy, 219-225
   maintenance of, 251-254
   results of, 270-271
   focal to major motor seizures induced
    by startling and nonspecific
    sound, 54
   major motor seizures evoked by
    specific and nonstartling sounds,
    57-59
   nature of sound, 44-45 (Table)
   nonspecific sounds, 45-54
   seizures evoked by nonspecific and
    and startling voices, 59-60
   seizures evoked by specific and
    startling sounds, 54-57
   specific sounds, 54-59
   startle as factor, 170

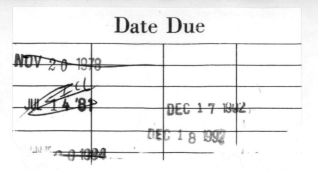